C000163751

of Nursing

Pediatric
Diagnostic
Procedures

Pediatric Diagnostic Procedures

With Guidelines for Preparing Children for Clinical Tests

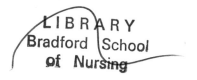

SUSAN COLVERT DROSKE, R.N., M.N.
Assistant Professor
School of Nursing
The University of Texas at Arlington
Arlington, Texas

SALLY A. FRANCIS, M.S., M.A.
Children's Medical Center of Dallas and Department of Pediatrics
The University of Texas Health Science Center at Dallas
Dallas, Texas

A WILEY MEDICAL PUBLICATION
JOHN WILEY & SONS
New York • Chichester • Brisbane • Toronto

Library of Congress Cataloging in Publication Data:

Droske, Susan Colvert.
    Pediatric diagnostic procedures.

    (A Wiley medical publication)
    Includes index.
    1. Children—Diseases—Diagnosis. 2. Children
—Medical examinations. 3. Pediatric nursing.
I. Francis, Sally A., joint author. II. Title.
[DNLM: 1. Diagnosis—In infancy and childhood.
2. Child, Hospitalized. WS141 D787p]
RJ50.D76   618.92′0075   80-22920
ISBN 0-471-04928-X

Printed in the United States of America

10 9 8 7 6 5 4 3 2 1

With love and thanks to my husband, Terry.
S.C.D.

To Alma Francis and Goldie Little, with love.
S.A.F.

Contributors

Linda C. Hoot, R.N., M.N.
Assistant Professor
Texas Woman's University
College of Nursing
Dallas, Texas

Paula Dimmitt, R.N., B.S.
Patient/Parent Educator
Children's Medical Center
Dallas, Texas

Foreword

For many years, the importance of the psychological aspects of child development has been appreciated, but not until recently have the psychological impact of hospitalization and the potential psychological trauma of diagnostic procedures on children been fully realized. Most pediatric nursing texts include only general information about diagnostic procedures, and they usually do not discuss any special considerations regarding the developmental stages. This book incorporates the developmental stages while providing specific information about the most commonly used diagnostic procedures in pediatrics for each body system. The categorization of the procedures by body systems and the use of a consistent format, with special attention to specific postprocedural assessments to detect possible complications, make this book a valuable contribution to the pediatric nursing literature.

Pediatric Diagnostic Procedures has been prepared for the practicing pediatric nurse as well as for the professional nursing student who is acquiring knowledge and developing skills and attitudes toward providing individualized, quality pediatric care. The use of this book is not confined to the hospital setting. It lends itself to a variety of health care settings such as day surgery, community health settings, clinics, child life programs, doctors' offices, or wherever a child enters the health care delivery system and is a candidate for a diagnostic procedure. This book can also serve as a beneficial resource in staff development.

The meaning, purpose, and value of parent-child teaching are stressed, with each developmental stage receiving the special consideration it deserves. The role of the nurse as a teacher and provider of quality health care is emphasized. The specific background information provided about each procedure sets the stage for selecting age-appropriate teaching, giving anticipatory guidance, and imparting predictable expectancies. Patient education by health care providers is becoming increasingly emphasized. Preoperative and preprocedure teaching is as beneficial to the child as it has proven to be with the adult. With the advent of television, the "normal" fears of childhood have been vivified; and because young children have difficulty in differentiating fact from fantasy, it becomes vitally important for adults to assist children by holding up reality when children are subjected to situations that may be damaging to their psychological development. The teaching of predictable expectancies, knowing what is going to happen, reduces the element of surprise and the feeling of having been deceived or taken advantage of. Energy wasted by children in attempting to cover up these feelings can thus be freely directed toward the development of a healthy personality. This book serves the function of child advocate.

In practice, the authors, Susan Droske and Sally Francis, are dedicated child advocates. Ms. Droske is a competent pediatric nurse and nurse educator; Ms. Francis is a child development practitioner and educator. I share my colleagues' philosophy that children are our greatest investment in the future and have a right to the finest health care possible. This book serves as an excellent guide to making this philosophy a reality.

Inez L. Teefy Ravell
Associate Professor of Nursing
Texas Woman's University
College of Nursing
Dallas Center
Dallas, Texas

Preface

Children are different from adults. Acknowledged in theory, this statement is not always carried out in practice. The difference, arising from the physical and psychological immaturity of children, demands our attention when diagnostic procedures are to be performed. Rarely, if ever, are adults placed in restraints, wildly kicking and biting, as a group of health care providers attempt a venipuncture. Yet this is not an uncommon occurrence with children. The psychological, social, and intellectual development of children does not always afford them the ability to tolerate unknown and/or intrusive procedures without a great deal of support. Children's ability to understand, accept, and cooperate with health care procedures is different from the adult's ability. Additionally, the physical immaturity of children dictates that medication dosage, positioning, use of restraints, interpretation of findings, and other factors involved in diagnostic procedures are altered when the patient is a child.

Because of these factors, we felt a need to assist children, as well as health care providers who interact with children, by writing a text on pediatric diagnostic procedures that focuses on both the physical and emotional needs of children undergoing these procedures. Our aim is to

prepare health care providers to carry out these procedures in such a way that the medical and nursing functions
can be integrated with a process of emotional preparation
and support for the child.

This text explains the most commonly performed diagnostic procedures in pediatrics; information the nurse will
need to plan, understand, and carry out in the procedures
is presented along with information about what the child
will see, hear, feel, and be expected to do. A process of
preparation is developed that can be applied to any child
undergoing any diagnostic procedure. This process, when
combined with the information about the procedure, can
enable nurses and all other health care providers to give
skilled physical and emotional support to children.

The authors are aware of the valuable contribution
made by both men and women in the health care professions and have tried to eliminate all sexist language from
the text. For clarity and simplicity, however, the feminine
pronoun has been used in reference to the health care
provider. To strike a balance, the masculine pronoun has
been used when mentioning the child.

We hope you will be able to build on the information
and ideas we have shared in this book from our study of
others' work and research and from our clinical experiences. We have learned from many clinicians and research-
ers. Equally important, we have learned from children
and their families. As you use this text in your clinical
setting, we hope you, too, will gain the satisfaction that
comes with preparation for diagnostic procedures, both
from your own preparation and from the preparation that
you provide to children.

S.C.D.
S.A.F.

Acknowledgments

This book represents the concern, support, and encouragement of many friends, colleagues, and family members.

We are grateful to those who reviewed portions of our manuscript and offered thoughtful criticism and suggestions: James R. Colvert, M.D., David Davis, M.D., Richard Srebro, M.D., Shannon Singer, R.N., M.S., and Charles Mann, M.D.

We are particularly indebted to Mary Clare Strub, R.N., M.S., and Inez Teefy Ravell, R.N., M.S., who patiently and thoroughly reviewed the final manuscript.

We appreciate the help of Carol Jacobs and Virginia Helton, who carefully typed the manuscript, and Kathy Quick, for her assistance.

We would like to thank Lewis E. Calver for the preparation of the original illustrations and Mike McCadden for the photographs.

We are grateful for the support and patience of Beverly Hudson and Nicki Capoziello Disbro.

Finally, we are indebted to Terry Droske for his unfailing patience and encouragement.

S.C.D.
S.A.F.

Contents

CHAPTER **6**
NEUROLOGIC DIAGNOSTIC PROCEDURES
113

CHAPTER **7**
GASTROINTESTINAL DIAGNOSTIC PROCEDURES
137

Pediatric
Diagnostic
Procedures

1

Preparation for Diagnostic Procedures: A Process for Mastery

WHY PREPARATION?

The preparation for diagnostic procedures is a process in which the health care provider, the child, and the family interact to promote the child's well-being in health care experiences. Diagnostic procedures are essential to maintaining or regaining health in children. These procedures provide the basic information the health care team must have to plan the child's care. These essential procedures present a conflict for the child and family, as well as for the health care provider. For the child and family, the procedure may be an unknown and consequently a frightening prospect. The health care provider can be troubled by the knowledge that diagnostic procedures can be uncomfortable, frightening, or painful for the children. The conflict that arises from "hurting while helping" can be difficult to resolve.

The resolution of this conflict for the health care provider can come from preparation for diagnostic procedures. The health care provider's preparation to participate in the procedures can ensure that the technical aspects of the procedure will go as smoothly as possible. This is to the child's benefit and comfort. Also, the health care provider will more effectively get the information needed to promote the child's health and well-being. When health care providers give emotional support to the child and family, they help the child master the difficult experience. Through such assistance, the benefits of the procedure are maximized; the child is emotionally, as well as physically, supported by health care.

It is unrealistic to hope that the stress of diagnostic

procedures can be eliminated. Rather, the health care provider can hope to help the child cope successfully with the stressful experience of diagnostic procedures. All people experience stress sometime in their lives. People who have successfully mastered difficulties before are more likely to succeed when confronting another stress. A health care experience such as a diagnostic procedure presents an opportunity to help the child cope with future stress experiences either in health care or in the child's world of home, school, and community.

Research and clinical practice show that the potential for psychological upset is inherent in a child's experience with health care. Immediate disturbances in behavior can continue and interfere with the child's usual development. If the child is not assisted in coping, the benefits of health care may be lessened and the disturbance created may outweigh the benefits. This potential is present because diagnostic procedures are usually unfamiliar experiences that involve discomfort and pain; consequently, they lead to fear and anxiety. Diagnostic procedures do not occur in a vacuum. They are a part of a total health care experience whether in the physician's office, a clinic, or a hospital. Emotional upset in one part of the total experience, such as trauma resulting from a diagnostic procedure, adds to the overall upset and has the potential for short or long-lasting trauma. In some instances, the trauma could interfere with the child's developmental progress. No matter what the upset, it could interfere with successful coping in future health care experiences.

Since the 1950s, because of the potential for psychological upset, ways of helping children cope with health care experiences have been studied through research and practice. Preparation, letting the child know what to expect, has been identified as one means of reducing potential upsets. Unfortunately, the importance of preparation is not always shown in practice. Perhaps this lack of preparation is due to the adults' fear that the child will be more, rather than less, upset by knowledge of what will happen. However, children often become more frightened by what they imagine. Fantasies of the experience frequently are more anxiety-provoking than the truth. The predictable expectancies that preparation affords release energy the child can use in coping.

Besides the fear of creating anxiety in the children, health care providers often feel preparation will take more time than they as hurried, often harried professionals have. However, experience shows that a prepared child can be more cooperative, thereby allowing the procedure to go more smoothly and save time for everyone. Before health care providers will take the time to make preparation a priority in their work, they must be convinced it will be of value both to the children and to them as care givers. The best reinforcement for a care giver is the sight of a child cooperating rather than becoming terrified by the procedure. This cooperation can result from the advance preparation of the child for the diagnostic procedure.

Health care providers frequently do not prepare children for procedures because they may not know how to do so or they do not know exactly what the procedure involves. This insecurity can be allayed when the care providers understand both the process of preparation and what the child will experience during the procedure. The preparation process, described in the first section of the text, will serve as a guide for the best preparation of a child and family for diagnostic procedures. Details of what the child will experience and appropriate actions of care givers during commonly performed procedures are included in later sections.

PREPARATION: A PROCESS

It should be reassuring to the health care provider to know that a "cookbook" approach to preparation is not effective. There is no list of ingredients that will prepare a child for a given procedure. Every child is similar to, yet different from, other children the same age. Developmental theories and research studies provide a base from which to begin. Environmental factors, particularly the child's family, and individual influences of personality and temperament must be taken into account. The preparation of all 5-year-olds in the same manner, using the same words and techniques, is potentially harmful. For example, a child's use of denial as a coping mechanism must be anticipated so that preparation will enhance the child's coping rather than tear down defenses and increase anxiety. This planning is most effective when it is based on an assessment of the developmental, environmental, and individual influences affecting the child's ability to cope with the procedure. Research studies on the preparation of children for health care experiences delineate three components of preparation: planning for the development of trust, understanding what is involved, and mastery of the experience. These components make up the process of preparation. Planning for this process must be geared to the developmental, environmental, and personal influences on the child's ability to cope with such health care experiences as diagnostic procedures.

Trust

Trust developed by the child in health care refers to the formation of a therapeutic alliance with the person participating in the experience with the child. Before the diagnostic procedure occurs and before preparation information can be conveyed effectively, the person responsible for the preparation* must get to know the child and be viewed by the child as a person who can be relied on to be

---

*Often preparation is provided by a nurse. In some instances it is provided by others such as physicians or child-life/child-development specialists. For simplification, this person will be referred to as the preparator.

honest, supportive, and comforting. Studies of young children separated from the people they trusted showed that they were overwhelmed when faced with new experiences without this known, trusted figure. Unless the child has developed trust in the preparator, the words, information, and techniques employed for imparting information will have little effect. Attention that should be directed by the child to the preparation will, instead, be tied up in the child's fantasy and in the child's attempts to figure out who this person is and what she is going to do.

Even when a child is to have a diagnostic procedure that he has undergone several times before, preparation and development of trust must take place each time. For example, a new-to-the-child staff person attempts to perform a venipuncture. Because the child has undergone

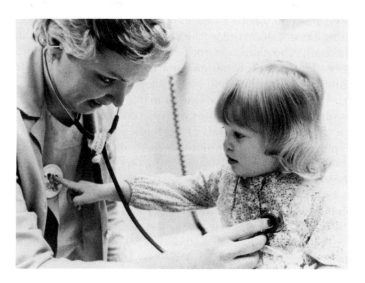

Figure 1-1
Trust, the formation of a therapeutic alliance, is essential to the process of preparation. Developing a positive relationship with a child is the first step in preparation.

this procedure before, and because the adult is pressed for time, the venipuncture is begun without the process of preparation. The child does not know this new person, nor does the adult have any information about the emotional or intellectual makeup of the child. Then the child loses control and becomes extremely agitated and difficult. The bewildered staff member cannot understand what is happening: "Why are you acting like this? You've had this done before. You know it will be over soon and won't be so bad if you hold still. What's wrong with you?"

What is wrong is the acutely felt lack of trust. The child has no way of knowing this person, no way of believing or trusting that this person has the child's best interest in mind. The adult, in turn, does not know the child. They have not formed an alliance. This is clearly seen in the adult's lack of knowledge of the rituals the child has come to associate with staying in control. In effect, the child has been presented with a new experience because the procedure has not occurred as the child had come to know it in the past. The child was not prepared for this new experience. The extra few minutes not taken to get to know the child, to allow the child to develop the confidence and trust that the experience can be manageable, has resulted in many more lost minutes of frustration and discomfort for the child and the staff. The child's anxiety and fantasy explanations for the unknown have interfered with his ability to maintain self-control and successfully cope with the diagnostic procedure.

Trust is the ingredient that allows us to share our feelings and fears with another person. This is as true for children as it is for adults. A person whom the child knows can spontaneously play and/or talk about the diagnostic procedure. A person not trusted by the child is likely to receive a "yes" or a nod of the head to any information or question. Many children who do not feel safe may appear to agree in hopes the adult will be pleased and satisfied and go away!

This therapeutic alliance, trust, must be established with the child's parents as well. The parents' level of anxiety is reflected in the child's anxiety. When parents feel secure and comfortable and have developed trust, they are better able to attend to the emotional needs of their child and to assist in the preparation process.

Developmental information shows that establishing trust with a 2-year-old is different from the manner in which one can establish trust with a 12-year-old. However, some guidelines apply to all children.

GUIDELINES FOR DEVELOPING TRUST

1. Trust must be established with the parent(s).

2. When meeting the parents for the first time and the child is present, introduce yourself to the parents and the child with a simple explanation of who you are and clearly state that you are not going to do anything to the child at this time. Tell them that you just want to talk and get to know them. Introduce yourself directly to the child and maintain eye contact with her. If the child is over four years of age, extend your hand for a handshake. A younger child may find the extended hand intrusive; older children may enjoy the "adultness" of the action and the physical contact provides a concrete beginning for establishing a relationship with you.

3. After introductions, talk directly to the parents. This begins your relationship with them and allows the child an opportunity to observe you in comfort without any expectations placed on her behavior.

4. If at all possible, it is helpful to be introduced to the family by a staff person, perhaps another nurse or physician whom the family knows and trusts. This allows for the transfer of positive feelings from their known figure to you.

5. Plan the first encounter so that you do not have to do anything to the child. Any physical experience that is intrusive into the child's body should, whenever possible, occur after the child knows you and has begun to establish trust in you.

6. When talking with the parents, keep the topic and

language used appropriate for the *child's* level of understanding. Even a young child, seemingly absorbed in play,
listens to the conversation of the adults. For example,
when telling the parents about an x-ray procedure that
will use dye, *dye* can be misinterpreted by the child to
mean *die*.

7. After talking with the parents, talk with the child.
This first conversation should not be about the preparation
for the procedure. Express interest in the child as a person
with an individual identity, not just as a patient.

8. When talking with the child, be sure you are in a
comfortable line of sight for the child. Do not stand
looking down at a small child. Instead, kneel down to the
child's eye level.

9. Be aware of your body in relation to the child's. A
comfortable distance from the child is one that does not
invade his personal body space. Being too close to an
unknown, untrusted person can be intrusive and arouse
anxiety in the child. If you are wearing clothing with
pockets, keep your hands out of them so the child can see
you are not hiding any unpleasant surprises, such as a
needle and syringe.

10. After this initial interaction, leave the child and
family (even if only for a few minutes) before beginning
any preparation. This time provides them an opportunity
to process information about you and to recognize you
when you do return. This simple act of recognition gives
them a feeling of being in control, in contrast to their
previous encounter with you when they had no knowledge,
only fantasies, of who you were or what would happen
next.

Understanding

Understanding is grasping the nature, significance, or
explanation of something. Studies on the preparation of
children for medical events stress the importance of shar-

ing cognitive information about the event. To be effective, information used in the process of preparation should include what the child will see, hear, feel, and be expected to do. This information is best coupled with a simple explanation of why the diagnostic procedure is necessary. Further explanations should be based on the child's questions and on the child's ability and readiness to profit from any additional information.

For children up to about the age of 12, a new experience is most easily comprehended through experience with the information. Without an experience, the actions, feelings, and information symbolized by the spoken words may mean something far different to the child than was intended. It is unlikely that the interpretation of the symbols is the same for the child as for the preparator. For this reason it is necessary to plan an experience for the child as part of developing understanding.

Developmental knowledge provides information about what a child can understand and how information can be presented. Materials that show what the child will see, hear, feel, and be expected to do aid in concreteness and help prevent or clarify distortions and fantasies. Pictures, photographs, body outlines, coloring books, story books, and other visual techniques such as slide tape shows or films have been developed to assist in the child's understanding of medical events and diagnostic procedures. Some of these materials are available commercially. Some materials may be obtained from various health care agencies. If materials are not available, they can be developed using the actual scenes from the local environment (hospital, clinic, or office setting) and resources available to the health care setting. One resource for finding materials is the Association for the Care of Children in Hospitals (1).

The use of such three-dimensional tools as doll play, puppet play, or art media provides a valuable adjunct in preparation. Medical play using props of real instruments and paraphernalia that the child will see and feel coupled with dolls, stuffed animals, or puppets allows a concrete enactment of the procedure. During this play, the preparator and child can identify ways in which the child can behave appropriately. These behaviors and mechanisms for maintaining self-control can be rehearsed and practiced in play. Play in this manner also gives the child an avenue for self-expression; recurrent or obsessional themes or acts in the play can be an indication of particularly upsetting elements in the forthcoming procedure. This is the clue for the preparator to attend to this part of the experience, to think further of the meaning of the event to the child, to attempt further development of understanding, and to provide more reassurance.

Although developmental information gives the preparator a basis for planning the preparation, environmental and individual influences on the child's coping must also be taken into account. For example, the child who uses denial as a primary defense will become more upset, rather than less, if presented with too much information about an event perceived as threatening. Without his characteristic defense, the child can be overwhelmed with anxiety and become unable to attend to the preparation process; he is caught up in warding off the anxiety aroused by the preparation information.

The developmental, environmental and, individual influences on the child provide guidelines for what the child can understand as well as the appropriate amount, complexity, and timing of the presentation of this information.

GUIDELINES FOR DEVELOPING UNDERSTANDING

1. The preparator should know what the child will see, feel, hear, and be expected to do during the procedure and in any preliminary activity leading to the diagnostic procedure.

2. The preparator should assess the child's developmental level of functioning and gather information from the parent(s) about environmental factors affecting the child's ability to cope with stress. For instance, has anyone close to the family been recently hospitalized? Has the family experienced a loss, move, or death that has not been adequately mourned and assimilated? Information about the child as an individual should be obtained. How does the child usually handle new experiences? Does the child separate easily from the parents and form new relationships with other adults and children with little or no trouble? Does the child have a preferred name? Is the child right-handed or left-handed? This can influence the decision of placement of needles, so that the child's preferred hand can be free for self-care, feeding, and play. What words does the family and child use for body parts and functions? The assessment of the child is conducted using whatever method the preparator finds effective. What is most important is that an assessment is made. The preparation information is then given to the child based on the preparator's assessment of what information will help the child's understanding.

3. The preparator should prepare the parent(s). This preparation is most effective if conducted away from the child while the child is comfortably engaged in other activities. This permits the parents to ask questions freely and provides them time to become comfortable with the procedure. The parents, in turn, can be supportive of the child during the procedure.

4. Concrete visual and interactive experiences should be part of the preparation information. The choice of materials is based on the assessment of the child as well as on the knowledge of what the child will see, hear, feel, and particularly, be expected to do during the procedure.

5. The choice of location for the preparation, timing, and length of time the child is engaged in the preparation must be based on the assessment of the child. For example, can the child attend comfortably to the preparation information in his present environment (which is known to him), or can he move to a new room, a new environment (where preparation might normally be conducted) without disruption? Has the child a well-developed concept of time to know what is meant when told "Tomorrow [or "This afternoon," or "After you wake up"] the nurse will put a cloth on your arm that will feel cold and wet"? What is the average attention span for the child? The preparation and time to interact with the concrete materials must be planned to fit the child's ability to pay attention.

6. Mastery-in-advance should be planned. The preparator should let the child know the predictable responses to the procedure and how the staff expects the child to behave. The child and preparator can develop ways to achieve the desired behaviors and practice these behaviors in play rehearsals.

Mastery

Mastery is the final component of the process of preparation. Although planning for mastery extends to the time after the diagnostic procedure is completed, opportunities for the development of mastery must be part of the development of trust and understanding. To master is to be in control of oneself and one's environment. Without opportunities for mastery-in-advance, mastery during and after the procedure, the child cannot be considered emotionally prepared for the experience. Without opportunities for mastery, the child remains a passive victim, rather than a participant in the diagnostic procedure.

Mastery is an active involvement with an experience. It brings with it the realization that "I have tackled a hard problem, but I did it! I can do it again." This is the feeling that leads to the confidence to try again, to endure the next stress. With each health care experience, one opportunity to develop mastery serves as mastery-in-advance to future health care experiences. For example, successful coping with, and mastery of, a diagnostic procedure such as a cardiac catheterization serves as preparation for cardiac surgery, if surgery is needed. Mastery of the catheterization experience gives the child the self-confidence to believe that the surgery can be endured and coped with successfully. This mastery has been called *immunological;* it innoculates one for psychological emergencies (2). Successful coping with one stressful experience adds to the potential for successfully coping with the next stressful experience, whether it is health care related or not.

The child's attempt to master a stressful experience will occur unassisted. However, the stress of the event may be more than the child can cope with. The child's unassisted attempts to master may become obstacles to the diagnostic procedure (as well as possibly frightening). For example, one child found that if he screamed loudly enough, he would focus his attention on his voice. This diverted his attention from the pain of needles being inserted and allowed him to hold still, which was the behavior expected of him. Unfortunately, his mechanism was disconcerting to the staff because it increased their anxiety to the point that it affected their performance of the procedure. In medical play, alternative means for maintaining control by diverting his attention from the source of pain were identified, rehearsed, and then put into practice. The preparator served as his "coach" during the procedure to assist him in the new behavior. Mastery for this child included the active development and application of a mechanism for maintaining self-control during the procedure. After the procedure, he continued developing his sense of mastery through regaining control of his environment: he was able to make choices about what kind of bandage to place on his arm, where he would go after the procedure, and what play materials he would use. These simple choices gave him control and thereby aided his development of mastery.

This is mastery: the active participation by the child in developing a feeling of being in control of himself in his environment. Mastery is provided through the identification and practice of behaviors that can increase the child's sense of being in control during the diagnostic procedure and in the events leading up to it. Mastery can be reinforced by the regaining of control and the ability to make realistic choices that affect the child and his body during the procedure.

GUIDELINES FOR DEVELOPING MASTERY

1. An opportunity for mastery-in-advance should be provided during the imparting of preparation information. Mechanisms for coping with the procedure should be developed with the child. These mechanisms should be practiced in play rehearsals of the procedure if such play is appropriate for the child. (For some children, such rehearsals might add to their anxiety; this decision is based on the assessment of the needs of the individual child.)

2. During the procedure, the preparator should help the child perform the identified mechanisms for the appropriate behavior.

3. Whenever possible during the procedure, the child should be given an opportunity to make choices. When the child makes choices and they are implemented, the child has a sense of being in control that enhances mastery. A simple choice such as "Do you want this Band-Aid or that one?" gives ownership of the child's body back to the child by allowing the child to control what is done to his body. Even simple choices provide the child with a sense of control and a feeling of mastery.

4. As soon as possible after the procedure, the child should be encouraged and assisted in expressing the experience. This "playing out" of the experience allows for the clarification of fantasies, the integration of the new experience into the child's existing repertoire of experience, and again, it gives control back to the child.

5. The preparator should continue to visit the child whenever possible when the child visits the clinic or on the following days of the child's hospitalization. This provides for the maintenance of trust the child has developed in the preparator, and it gives the preparator the opportunity to observe the child's continual integration of the experience.

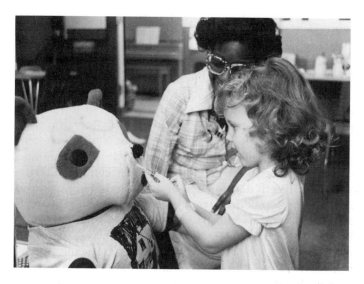

Figure 1-2
Play after diagnostic procedures provides opportunities for the young child to master the experience, to learn about instruments and events that were unknown and frightening. Concrete learning through play can effectively take place.

INFLUENCES ON THE CHILD THAT AFFECT PREPARATION

As stated earlier, every child is similar to, yet uniquely distinct from, other children the same age. Developmental understanding provides for the similarities among children. Environmental factors and individual influences of personality and temperament explain many diversities. Commonalities as well as individual differences among children must be considered when planning the process of preparation. The roles of trust, understanding, and mastery have already been explored. The importance of considering developmental, environmental, and individual factors must now be examined.

Developmental Influences

Developmental knowledge provides the basis from which to begin planning the preparation for a specific child. Cognitive development influences the manner, timing, and complexity of the presentation of information about what the child will see, hear, feel, and be expected to do. The ability and ease with which a child can establish trust depends on the level of his psychosocial development. Developmental knowledge also provides an understanding of the common fears and fantasies that children experience at different developmental stages and illuminates the normal developmental struggles facing the child to which health care and diagnostic procedures add an additional burden. Also the understanding of psychosocial development assists in planning for mastery, it helps the preparator determine the appropriate techniques to use in mastery-in-advance and in mastery during and after the procedure. For example, play with dolls is appropriate for a 3-year-old interacting with his parent and the preparator. Eight-year-olds receive support and information from peers. Preparation that allows for peer interaction can be appropriate and successful with this age group; however, it would be chaotic with 3-year-olds. For adolescents, explanations that involve a more abstract understanding may be appropriate.

Environmental Influences

There are many environmental influences on children. Those influences of particular importance in the process of preparation include: the family's environment, the family's functioning, the child's reactions to health care, the child's previous experiences with stress, and the child's role in the family. Families with limited health care experiences or who are undergoing disruption and stress may be less able to support the child's emotional needs during the experience of health care. This information is important; it aids the preparator plan for both the child's and the family's preparation, and it helps the family and the preparator understand each other's behavior.

Such previous life experiences as the child's experiences with separation, with loss, and with health care will influence a child's behavior. The environment of a child admitted to the hospital for a reevaluation of a corrected atrial septal defect will differ from that surrounding a child scheduled for a first catheterization to determine if there is a defect. The family's reactions will vary considerably and influence the child's level of anxiety. For the first family, the catheterization procedure may determine if the child can now participate in active sports. For the second family, fears of the unknown and the prospect of surgery based on the findings of the diagnostic procedure may greatly decrease their ability to give emotional support to their child.

The socioeconomic level and cultural influences of the family should be considered when planning the child's preparation. Economic restrictions may prevent the parents from staying with the child during extended procedures that would require time away from work. The child's anxiety level and ability to trust will then be influenced by the absence of his primary emotional support.

The child whose family uses English as a second language may respond to verbal instructions differently than a child whose first language is English. Cultural influences may be reflected in a general lack of trust in health care personnel, thereby making it more difficult for the child and parent to develop a therapeutic alliance with the preparator.

Individual Influences

In addition to developmental and environmental influences, the child as an individual will affect the preparation process and should be considered in the planning. The child's temperament, common patterns of defense, likes and dislikes can influence the manner in which the preparator establishes trust, presents the preparation information, and provides mastery activities. For example, one 8-year-old, described by his parents as an outgoing child who has adapted well to new experiences in the past, may use intellectualization as a primary defense and coping mechanism. This child may become absorbed in a story book provided to help the child understand the preparation information. After the procedure, the child may use intellectual skills to create stories about the procedure as a mastery device. Another child the same age may be described as shy around strangers and frequently uses regression as a means of coping with stress. The child's regression may be seen in an increased fear of separation from his parents. When preparation information is presented, both children should be prepared for what they would see, hear, feel, and would be expected to do in the procedure. However, the emphasis and focus of the preparation should vary to meet the individual needs of these two children. The first child should have ample opportunity to interact with the preparation information and to ask questions that will assist in the child's intellectual coping style. The second child should be told where he will be, where his parents will be, and when they will be reunited. The therapeutic alliance must be strong enough to allow this child to use the preparator as an emotional support in the absence of his parents.

SUMMARY

When preparation for diagnostic procedures is viewed as a process involving the development of trust, understanding, and mastery based on the developmental, environmental, and individual influences on the child, it provides guidelines for preparing any child for any diagnostic procedure. When the preparator knows what a child will see, hear, feel, and be expected to do in the procedure, this information can be presented to the child in ways that encourage the child's trust, understanding, and mastery. After establishing trust with the child, such preparation information as what the preparator knows the child will see, hear, feel, and be expected to do can be presented to help the child's understanding. The presentation of this information opens opportunities for a child to begin the process of mastery; the child can actively develop or regain control of himself in his environment.

The facilitated trust, understanding, and mastery helps the child cope with an experience that could cause undue physical and emotional stress. The resulting emotional preparedness does not take away anxiety. In fact, it may not reduce such visible signs of upset as crying; however, it does allow the child to engage in some anticipatory worry, to begin the process of self-control, to experience self-esteem and confidence, and to accept comfort from the health care providers.

Preparation is the process that the preparator must do before, during, and after a diagnostic procedure. Before the procedure, trust must be gained and understanding begun, so that mastery-in-advance can be developed through preparation information. During the procedure, trust is supported while the preparator assists the child in carrying out those behaviors previously identified as providing comfort, self-control, and cooperation. After the procedure, the preparator provides opportunities for the child to play or take part in conversation; these opportunities help the child integrate the experience and continue to master the procedure. This mastery can serve as mastery-in-advance for subsequent health care experiences.

REFERENCES

1. Association for the Care of Children in Hospitals, 3615 Wisconsin Avenue, NW, Washington, DC.
2. Kliman G: *Psychological Emergencies of Childhood.* New York, Grune and Stratton, Inc., 1968.

2

Preparing Children for Diagnostic Procedures

The judgment of knowing what to say to a child in preparation for a diagnostic procedure must be based on the developmental, environmental, and individual influences on the child's ability to cope with the stress of a diagnostic procedure. These influences will be different for each child in the guidance they provide for the development of trust and the facilitation of the child's understanding and mastery. However, developmental information in specific age groups can be helpful in planning for the child's needs, fears, and common fantasies based on the cognitive and affective processes available to the child.

When trust, understanding, and mastery are included in the preparation process, the child has an opportunity for emotional growth. With adequate preparation, threatening procedures can be emotionally beneficial for the child and can aid the child in coping with stress encountered not only in subsequent health care experiences but also in other areas of the child's life.

INFANTS

Infancy (birth to 24 months) is a phase of development in which the child is unfolding and developing dramatically. The developmental process in infancy is particularly important. The infant begins to develop coordination of simple sensorimotor skills and fundamental reflex actions. Experience with the environment initiated by fundamental reflex actions gradually builds the coordination of purposive motions. The end of this stage is marked when the infant begins to talk and achieves easy motor skills. Because the infant has limited, if any, word use and inadequate conceptual skills with which to prepare for a diagnostic procedure, preparation at this age can easily be overlooked. However, the infant should be provided with trust and mastery. For this reason, the parents are the primary focus of the preparation.

The establishment of basic trust or mistrust during these first two years of life could influence later development. The solution to this problem of trust lies in the consistency with which the infant's needs are attended. When the infant learns that he will not be left hungry, he will learn that the people and the environment can be trusted. Preparation that aids the parent(s) in feeling comfortable and secure enhances the parent's ability to respond to the infant's needs. Up to approximately six months of age, the infant will accept new and unknown care givers who are attentive to such cues as how to best hold, feed, and comfort the infant.

With the onset of "stranger anxiety," the infant is less likely to tolerate separation from the parent and handling by an unknown person. It is important to learn from the parent the particular actions that promote comfort and a sense of well-being. If the parents cannot be present during the diagnostic procedure, this information can be used to make the infant as comfortable as possible and to soothe and calm the child during and after the procedure.

Older infants, up to 24 months, understand the diagnostic procedure to be nothing more than pain, discomfort, and separation. Parents should be encouraged to bring familiar objects from home that can, whenever possible, remain with the child. These familiar objects are comforting to the infant. As soon as possible after the procedure, the infant should be returned to the parents; they can best relieve the anxiety aroused by the separation.

Infants who can crawl and walk should be encouraged to move around to release tension as soon as possible after the procedure. Mastery can be enhanced by such age-appropriate activity.

Thus, the preparation of infants for diagnostic procedures is the emotional preparation of the parents through facilitating the parents' trust, understanding, and mastery. With such assistance, the parents can better meet the emotional needs of their child. Information about the infant's personal preferences for comfort and soothing can be used to calm the child during the procedure. Motor activity as soon after the procedure as possible provides the child with discharge of tension and opportunities for mastery of the environment.

TWO- TO 4-YEAR-OLDS

The hallmark of 2- to 4-year-olds is the acquisition and rapid development of language skills. According to the Piaget theory, the child is in the cognitive stage of preconceptual thought. During these years the improvement of the child's verbal skills may cause the adult to overestimate the child's ability to understand the diagnostic procedure and benefit from verbal preparation. However, as the name of this stage implies, the child cannot think in concepts. Symbolic functions are being acquired; the child is beginning to retain mental pictures of objects and people. The word for the object can be mentally created without requiring the physical presence of the object.

This emerging cognitive development is seen in the child's increasing ability to be separated from his parents and in his ability to use transition objects or objects such as car keys to reassure him that his parents will return.

Before the onset of preconceptual thought, the infant's play in the physical world was exploratory. The practice of developing physical skills and then their use to bring about novel happenings in the environment constituted most play behavior. Now, with symbolization, play takes on a dramatic, make-believe quality. The child can reenact, through play, events that have occurred in the child's immediate experience. For example, a 3-year-old child is fascinated by, and can play with, doll houses that were enjoyed before for their physical nature: handling, throwing, making doorbells ring. It is not uncommon to observe children in this age group intently recreating health care experiences from their own perspective. Three-year-old Melissa was busily engaged in play with a hospital doll house. She moved the dolls in and out of the building. She then placed one in the ambulance. She looked at it, took it out, gave it a resounding spanking, and said "You've been bad, bad, bad. You have to go to the hospital!"

Melissa was reenacting her experience from her understanding and perspective. Children this age think egocentrically; the world is interpreted only as they experience it. The world would not be understood from another person's perspective; this requires thought the preconceptual child cannot manage. From Melissa's perspective, hospitalization was punishment. Her only experiences before hospitalization with pain inflicted by other persons were when she was corrected with swats on her hands or bottom by her mother and father. Now she was experiencing pain from others, so she believed she must have been bad. This pain was punishment not unlike that of her parents. Through play she was able to symbolically share what she thought was happening. Her play provided an opportunity for the preparator to clarify and reassure her that she had not been bad, that she had not done anything to cause the pain. It also provided an opportunity to share information with the parents about how children commonly interpret health care experiences. With this knowledge, they were able to comfort Melissa.

Because of the child's egocentrism and immature thought processes, reality and fantasy are closely intertwined. The child's fantasy can be as real for the child as reality. Thus, many of the child's attempts to relate to the world are illogical. Melissa's understanding is illogical to an adult's way of thinking; of course she is not being punished. The health care team has to help her deal with what is real to her. She needs simple, concrete explanations as to why she must be hurt, coupled with a great deal of comfort and reassurance about the procedure. The child's fantasy must be taken seriously. It is only when the preparator understands the child's fantasy that reality can become reassuring. Often the child's fantasy is more upsetting. When the reality can be presented, the fantasy takes on more realistic dimensions, becomes more manageable and less anxiety-provoking.

The knowledge of these misconceptions is helpful in understanding the child's attempts to master a stressful experience such as a diagnostic procedure. Understanding also helps the preparator encourage the child's trust, understanding, and mastery. One such misconception is termed *animism;* that is, inanimate objects having lifelike properties attributed to them by the child in the same sense that people are alive and active. These inanimate objects have, according to the child, feelings and the ability to act on their own volition. Animism can be seen in the child's protectiveness of a favorite doll or teddy bear brought from home. The favored object should not be used in demonstrations of preparation information; if the child has attributed feeling to the doll, the anxiety evoked in the child at the possibility of the doll having an injection will be very real. Injections are painful to the child; therefore, they must hurt the doll. Animism coupled with the indistinct boundaries between fantasy and reality make the child particularly vulnerable to misinterpretation of information. The preparator must remember how easily fantasy can become alarming to the child. Attention should be paid to understanding the child's fantasy explanations for the events he is encountering. The fantasy should be clarified and grounded with reality to aid the child's management of fears.

Imminent justice is another quality of egocentric thought in children at this developmental level of cognition. Imminent justice is the assumption that the world is equipped with a built-in system of law and order. This is readily seen when asking children why they have to get shots; the common response is "because I was bad."

Another common misconception is *artificialism*. This is the notion that everything in the world, all objects and events, are designed by people. These two concepts, imminent justice and artificialism, point out the need to continually reassure the child that he has not been bad and is not being subjected to health care experiences as punishment. To help the child understand, the child needs to be reassured that he is in the hospital or clinic to fix something specific. These are concrete examples that can be understood, and they convey to the child the fact that discomforting health care experiences are necessary and are not concocted at the whim of the adults.

Because the child's concept of time is limited, preparation should not be conducted too far in advance of the procedure. Since children at this stage can only conceptualize those things they have experienced, preparation information that aids understanding must be limited, unless the child has experienced the event. However, understanding and mastery acquired through medical play and rehearsal of needed behaviors can provide information for which the child has no previous experience.

Preparation should emphasize the end of the event and some pleasurable event that will take place afterward. This helps the child, who cannot judge the passing of time, to realize that the experience will end. Planning during the preparation for something after the procedure helps the child understand that there will be an end. The plan may be something the preparator and child can discuss during the diagnostic procedure if the child is awake. This can provide a calming influence for the child. For example, the child may plan to go with her father to the coffee shop. In play, the preparator and child can enact the scene of the child leaving the diagnostic procedure, joining a "daddy doll," and going to a coffee shop. This play can be repeated several times; the doll might even be taken to the procedure so that "daddy doll" can remind the child that the experience will end and she will be rewarded.

In psychosocial development, the child begins to acquire a sense of autonomy rather than shame and doubt. This implies that the child is rapidly acquiring a sense of separateness from his primary emotional support, usually the mother. However, the child's reaction to the stress of a new, strange environment is frequently seen in the child's regression. For this reason, the parents continue to be a primary focus in preparation. Parents should be prepared for procedure separately from the child so they can freely talk, question, and explore their own feelings about the event. This preparation will help them be supportive of the child during the child's preparation.

Familiar objects from home and transition objects are commonly used by children in this group for comfort and support, particularly transition objects. The transition object symbolizes the security of the primary emotional support figure. The identification of this object and having it available to the child during the procedure, if at all possible, helps the child cope with the separation and stress of this new experience.

At this stage of psychosocial development, the child is acquiring a sense of autonomy. In order for this to happen, the child must learn body control. Experiences that threaten the evolving sense of autonomy pose particular difficulty for the child. Virtually every health care experience is a threat to autonomy. Efforts to assist mastery should be guided by the realization that the child needs positive experiences in the control of his body. Children this age often view their bodies as containers for bones and fluids. A puncture is particularly threatening because it might, in the child's view, result in a hole from which one's insides could leak out. It is no wonder Band-Aids are so important to young children and should be taken seriously by the preparator.

Mastery following the procedure is most important to this age child, since cognitive limitations may prevent development of true understanding before the actual experience occurs. The procedure can be sorted out and understood in play, afterward. Opportunities for the child to play after the procedure in the presence of a staff member can help the child achieve mastery. During this postprocedure play, the preparator can clarify incorrect and fearful fantasies and thus enhance the child's mastery.

Guidelines for Preparing 2- to 4-Year-Olds

1. From a developmental perspective, remember, the child's verbal skill does not, as yet, signify conceptual, cognitive ability. Fantasy and reality are closely related in the child's experience. Since the child can call on little previous experience to provide him with mental images, words used in preparation information should be those used by the child and family to denote body parts and functions. Words should be used as concretely and unambiguously as possible. The child has newly acquired sense of individuality and is struggling to determine a sense of autonomy. Stress may result in a regression to earlier, more secure levels of functioning. This should be accepted and supported. When the child is ready, progress to the previous level of functioning can begin.

2. From an environmental perspective, the child's regression, coupled with the parents' level of comfort or anxiety, influences the child's ability to develop trust and to absorb the preparation information. For these reasons, parents are an important focus in the preparation. Parents should be prepared separately from the child so that the child cannot misconstrue words used in the parents' preparation and in their questions to the preparator.

3. From an individual perspective, the child's use of play can serve as an appropriate vehicle for understanding the unique, fantasy explanations the child may have for the experience. Concrete play experiences are particularly important in helping this age child develop mastery after the procedure. Whereas before the procedure, the child had little experience to call on to symbolize the experience, the child now has experienced the procedure and needs an opportunity to "play out" the experience in the presence of a staff member who is alert to clues of misconceptions and fantasies.

4. Play experiences should be readily available to help the child move beyond regression to reestablish the child's developing autonomy.

5. The 2- to 4-year-old child's development of trust,

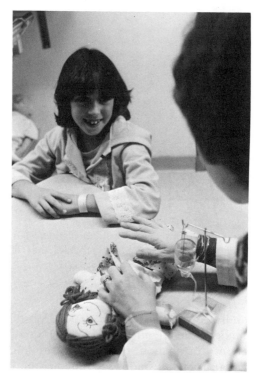

Figure 2-1(a)

Research has shown sensation preparation to be effective. The use of tangible objects in preparation that the child will feel and see during the procedure provides a concrete experience necessary to the child's development of understanding.

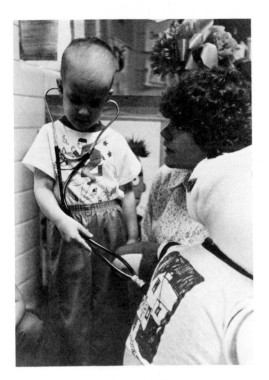

Figure 2-1(b)
Medical play using props of real instruments increases the child's understanding of the procedure and provides the child with an avenue for self-expression.

understanding, and mastery will depend on the parent's level of anxiety; the attention to the provision of concrete, unambiguous information; the use of transition objects to provide comfort if the child is separated from the parents during tbe procedure; and the use of play to understand the procedure, to work through tbe anxiety and fantasy aroused by the experience, and to enhance autonomy and mastery.

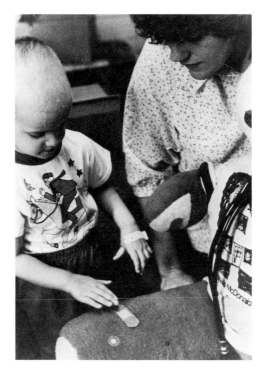

Figure 2-2
Preplay and postplay experiences provide an opportunity for the child to rehearse expected behaviors and play out disturbing feelings aroused by the diagnostic procedure. The presence of the preparator assists both the child's understanding and the child's trust and mastery.

FOUR- TO 7-YEAR-OLDS

Children in the 4- to 7-year-old group have had more experiences that can be used by the child and the preparator. Although language has developed to the point that the child expresses thoughts in sentences, the ease with which all thought can be expressed is far from the adult's ability. Play continues to be an important vehicle for self-expression. Play also continues to be a significant method through which the child learns about his world. Play can be particularly effective for the child whose verbal skills are not yet refined. This age child is in the phase of intuitive thought: the child's thinking is based on immediate perceptions and experiences rather than on mental operations. What he sees is what he perceives, and his understanding of a situation is often limited to the information he has on hand. The child continues to be egocentric. The world revolves around him and he is unable to mentally assume the position of another. This egocentrism changes as the child adds more and more experiences from his physical and social world. Two aspects of intuitive thought that bear on the child's preparation are centering and transductive reasoning.

The term *centering* refers to a tendency of the child to concentrate on a single characteristic of an object while excluding its other features. Because of very selective attention, the child's understanding of the object could be distorted. This type of thinking could influence the child's view of instruments to be used on his body during a procedure. Consequently, it is important to include three-dimensional experiences in the preparation information. The child needs to handle objects that he may see and feel during the procedure. Pictures can acquaint the child with the object, but the child's perception of the object can be distorted, inappropriate, or inadequate for his understanding. In some cases, the distortion can add to the child's fears and fantasies about what will be done to him during the procedure. By handling objects, playing with them, incorporating them in rehearsal of expected behaviors, the child has an opportunity to learn about the object. During such play, the preparator has an opportunity to observe distortions and offer clarification.

Another characteristic of intuitive thought is the child's reasoning ability; it is neither deductive nor inductive, rather *transductive*. The child goes from particular to particular without looking for similarities between them. An example is seen in the child's inference that the physician who enters the room is coming for him instead of one of the other children in the room. The child was here earlier and the doctor came to get him so, here is a doctor, he must be coming to get him. It is interesting to watch the responses of children when health care providers enter a hospital playroom. If the individual is easily identified, that is, if he has on a white coat, all of the young children freeze. The apprehension with which every child watches shows that they fear he has come for them specifically.

In psychosocial development the child in the 4- to 7-year-age group is faced with acquiring a sense of initiative and overcoming a sense of guilt. This child has fully separated his identity from his primary emotional support, usually his mother, and is able to tolerate separations for extended periods of time, even days. Conscious control of his body has also been developed and he is able to more fully participate in his environment. This freedom is seen in the child's initiative. He is busy, constantly undertaking new play and exploring new experiences. However, this initiative brings the child into conflict with the initiative and needs of others. This conflict is the source of guilt the child feels. A common example is the child who feels he is being subjected to health care procedures as a punishment for having played outside when his mother had told him not to.

Specific anxieties about health care have been found to be reflected at certain developmental stages. Four- and 5-year-olds fear the experience. Five- and 6-year-olds express more fear of strangeness and unfamiliarity of the setting; 7-year-olds' anxiety arises more from their fear of loss of control and fear of body mutilations.

Establishing trust with children in this group is easier and accomplished in shorter periods of time than with younger children. Trust, the therapeutic alliance, takes on increased significance for the child who now sees himself as a separate individual. The preparator can fully use the child's ability to trust both during preparation and to strengthen support during the procedure. Establishing trust with the parents continues to be vital since the degree of anxiety they experience is reflected in the child's behav-

Preparation information that increases the child's understanding must be presented within the range of the child's cognitive abilities. What the child will see, hear, feel, and be expected to do should be presented in ways that take into account centering and transductive reasoning. For example, if the child will be expected to breathe deeply with a mask over his face, the child should have an opportunity to handle the mask, to explore all of its traits to avoid focusing on one aspect of it that might be distorted and arouse additional fantasies and fears during the procedure. This presentation of preparation information can be accomplished in play that uses the real equipment that the child will see and feel, as well as through dolls, stuffed animals, or puppets. The identification of expected behaviors can be enacted by the preparator with a doll, then the child and preparator together can develop means for the child's accomplishment of the behavior.

During the procedure the preparator can help the child carrying out the behavior mechanism that was developed. If the stress of the experience is still overwhelming and the child is not very successful in carrying out the expected behaviors, the preparator should not shame the child by saying something like, "You said you were going to count to 10 and hold your arm still. You're not holding still! You're not doing what you said!" Instead, the preparator should offer other means to assist the child in holding still and not increase the child's guilt and sense of failure. "You're really trying hard and doing well. I know how hard it is. Keep up the good work." These phrases can give the child support.

After the procedure, the child can be complimented on his ability to do whatever he was able to do. This positive interchange reinforces what the child was able to do without adding to the child's sense of failure. The reinforcement can be continued in play after the procedure. "Playing out" of stressful events continues to be important for children in this age group. It is in this postprocedure play that the child can fully experience a sense of mastery, of having survived a very difficult experience.

SEVEN- TO 11-YEAR-OLDS

Seven- to 11-year-olds are in a distinct phase of development. They have acquired the ability to think and reason logically. This phase of development is called the phase of concrete operations. The child's thought is operational, and consequently experience can be ordered and related to an organized whole. Although children at these ages are not able to think abstractly, their thought processes more closely resemble those of adults. This development greatly facilitates the child's understanding of the preparation information. Fantasy loses its strong hold on the child's thought and reality is based more on the child's developing mental operations. This in turn enables him to understand and anchor experience in an orderly, logical, and communicative system. During these years, thought shifts from inductive to deductive reasoning. The child also develops a full understanding of the concept of time.

Within psychosocial theory, the child in these years acquires a sense of industry while overcoming a sense of inferiority. Although the family was his primary environment, he has now entered school and his peers become important influences. The child is learning about himself in relation to other children; he asks himself, "What can I do? What can they do? Can I do what they can?"

Competition becomes important as evidenced by an increasing interest in organized group games. Competition in play provides a means for sorting out who the child is in relation to other children. The comparisons, judgments, and competition aid the child in developing a sense of competence. This sense of competence is the resolution of the developmental conflict, industry vs. inferiority. It leaves him feeling that he can do things, make things, and achieve.

Although the world of peers takes on equal or even greater importance than the child's relationships with adults, establishing trust with children in this age group is easily accomplished when one is straight forward, honest, and accepting of the child. The therapeutic alliance can be particularly helpful in bulwarking the child in times of stress. During the diagnostic procedure, the child in this group may have high expectations for his behavior that he cannot fulfill. For example, he may feel that it is babyish to cry, yet tears come. Knowing that one of the adults involved will accept this "weakness" without harshly judging him provides the support the child needs to cope. This support is not seen as reassurance if given by someone the child does not know and with whom he has not formed a trusting relationship. Reassurance from an unknown person is frequently misconstrued as condenscension and adds to the child's feeling of inferiority and/or failure.

Because children in this age group possess a greater attention span than before, preparation information can now be shared in a process that allows for more time. The child's concept of time is such that the preparation can be spread out over a period of time or conducted a few days ahead of time without arousing unusual anxiety. For some children, preparation information shared a day or two ahead provides them with the opportunity to exercise their advanced cognitive skills. They can think about the procedure and develop questions about it. However, the timing of the preparation information must always be based on the assessment of the child. From a developmental viewpoint, the child may be able to profit from timing that allows him to think about the information and ask questions. From an individual perspective, the child may be overwhelmed by the health care experience and express his anxiety in regression. Advance preparation might provide too long a time for the child to think about the procedure and could actually increase anxiety rather than reduce it.

Preparation information should continue to focus on what the child will see, hear, feel, and be expected to do. Caution must be taken not to make the explanation for why the procedure is scheduled too complex. An explanation based on physical causation is most appropriate. Because the child is not yet able to think abstractly, this explanation should include body outlines, pictures, or models to illustrate the explanation.

The child still must learn first in the physical world, then use his mental operations to apply the learning to himself and his problem-solving. For this reason, it is good to continue using three-dimensional, concrete activities in preparation information. What is different now, again based on the individual preferences of the child, is the use of dolls and doll play. Not infrequently, older children in this group, 9- to 11-year-olds, will resist the dolls and accept them only when they are used distinctly as models. Yet after the diagnostic procedure the child will readily engage in medical play using the dolls as younger children do. It is as though initially the child tries very hard to establish himself as all that he should be. It is only after the experience and its threat is over that self-control can be relaxed and the child allows himself to fully explore all the feelings evoked by the experience.

Peers can play a role in the preparation process. Preparing two children together in this age group may be beneficial. They form an alliance with one another that can be supportive and can assist them in talking about and processing the information. The use of peer support must be based, again, on the assessment of the child's development. Children in this age group tend to view health experiences as threats to their sense of competency. They fear body mutilation and loss control. However, these fears may be so pronounced that a peer involved in their preparation might increase the child's fear of loss of control and of being judged as less capable by the peer. Such increased anxiety would interfere with the child's attention to the preparation information.

The preparator can discuss the behaviors that will be expected of the child and rehearse with him the mecha-

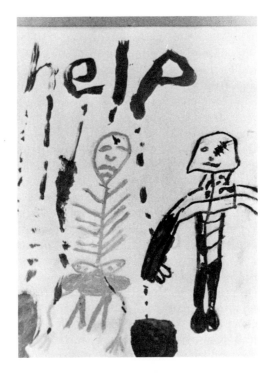

Figure 2-3

Fear of body mutilation is shared by many children. Expressions of feelings, such as those expressed in artwork, provide insight into how best to prepare a child.

nism for control. Children in this group are more likely to use skills they have rather than choosing to use the preparator as the prime means for maintaining control. Younger children frequently identify with holding hands with the preparator and squeezing hands tightly when a painful event occurs. Children in the concrete operations group more frequently decide to count from 25 backward or to count in another language they are learning in school. Not only does this help them maintain control, it also allows them to show off competency. The recognition of success, or even of partial success, helps the child overcome the pull toward inferiority and enhances the child's sense of mastery.

In the preparation information, simple analogies can now be made for the child that can help him understand. Analogies are particularly helpful if they can be demonstrated concretely.

Individual coping patterns can be used, particularly after the procedure, to enhance the child's mastery. A child who uses intellectualism as a coping pattern can be encouraged to write stories about the experience or make a tape recording that tells about the procedure. He can be encouraged to illustrate his account of the event with pictures by him or perhaps with photographs taken with a Polaroid camera. This exercise serves as a means for "playing out" the experience just as doll play does for other children. The stories can be read together by the preparator and child, giving an opportunity for the preparator to clarify misconceptions and for the child to ask further questions. These stories and artwork should be displayed in the office or on the hospital ward. This is public acclamation that the child has endured a difficult experience. It provides public recognition of the child's ability and mastery and adds to the child's feelings of self-esteem and mastery. Not all children, particularly the younger ones in this group, will be as able to use intellectual skills in mastery experiences after the procedure. Consequently, provisions for medical play opportunities are important to help the child understand the experience and work through its puzzling elements. Mastery is, of course, enhanced when the child is allowed to make realistic choices before, during, and after the procedure. These choices give the child a feeling of being in control, even if in only a small way. Provision for choices also allows the child to continue to see himself as a capable person, able to have an effect on her environment. This is particularly important for the child who fears a loss of control and who has feelings of inferiority.

ADOLESCENTS

Adolescence marks the onset of mature thought processes. This developmental phase of cognition is referred to as the phase of formal operations. The adolescent's thought represents the integration of all past intellectual operations. Thought now becomes abstract, not limited to the physical experience. The actual experience of an event is not necessary for the adolescent's understanding. Hypothetical problems and solutions can be considered. The adolescent can think about the past, the present, and the future. The adolescent can confront a problem, formulate a number of possible answers, and explore them as possible solutions. Reasoning at this level is both inductive and deductive. Because of these advances in thought, the adolescent is able to theorize about the world and mentally explore various possibilities without losing the sense of reality.

Psychosocial theory describes the adolescent's task of identity formation as the acquisition of a sense of identity while overcoming a sense of identity diffusion. The adolescent is concerned with determining who he is, what he can be, and what his body can do. These determinations are expressed by Erikson in the conflicts of perspective versus time diffusion, self-certainty versus apathy, role experimentation versus negative identity, anticipation of achievement versus work paralysis, sexual identity versus bisexual diffusion, leadership versus authority diffusion, and ideological polarization versus diffusion of ideals (1). Each of these conflicts is important to the understanding of the sometimes contradictory behaviors of adolescents and in the consideration of the implications of diagnostic procedures. For example, the adolescent can comprehend why a procedure is scheduled and contemplate the implications of the outcome. A cardiac catheterization may result in a reevaluation of the adolescent's physical activities and may warrant new restrictions on physical activities. The hypotheses and possible outcomes the adolescent is now capable of considering may heighten the conflict of identity formation. If restrictions are imposed, self-certainty, role and work exploration, and sexual identity conflicts may add to the adolescent's anxiety about the upcoming procedure.

The adolescent's mature reasoning abilities influence the process of preparation. Trust, the formation of a therapeutic alliance, continues to be important, particularly now that the adolescent is moving beyond the immediate family and is attempting to establish a separate identity. A trusted adult can serve as a role model as well as a source of guidance and support during the diagnostic health care experience. Preparation information is presented differently than with younger children. The information can begin with the reason for the procedure and proceed to the concrete details involved. Explanations can be given that involve abstract understanding. The use of body outlines and pictures can be used as an aid to understanding but are not essential as with younger children. Three-dimensional activities are not necessary now, since the adolescent can understand the information.

It is still important to prepare the adolescent for what he will see, hear, feel, and be expected to do. However, this information can be coupled with explanations of why and how these events fit into a logical overall process. The adolescent will need the preparator to help him identify the expected behaviors and explore ways in which he can carry out these behaviors. It is important to reassure the adolescent that if he should lose control and become visibly upset and cry, the staff will not find the behavior unusual. The adolescent should be reassured ahead of time that crying is a usual response to discomfort and is not interpreted by the preparator or staff as a sign of the adolescent's failure.

Because adolescents can hypothesize, consider several alternatives, and think them through to a logical conclusion, they need more time to think about the information that has been presented. The preparator needs to remain available to the adolescent so that when the adolescent formulates questions, he can discuss them with the preparator.

When presenting the preparation information, the preparator needs to keep in mind that the older the adolescent, the easier it will be for him to understand. Young adolescents, when dealing with the stress of the diagnostic procedure, may regress to earlier levels of thought, and it is important that an assessment be made of the individual influences on the adolescent's coping ability. If the preparator is unsure how best to present preparation information to the young adolescent, it is wise to present the information as one would to a child in the concrete operations phase of cognitive development. The concrete materials and three-dimensional activity explaining the information will be easily understood. As the adolescent gains control over his anxiety, additional explanations requiring abstract thought can be added.

Mastery is as important for adolescents as for younger children. The adolescent frequently wavers between feeling self-confident and capable and feeling apathetic and ineffective. Providing opportunities for the adolescent to make realistic choices assists him in feeling in control of his body at a time when his body seems out-of-control.

Mastery can be enhanced after the procedure through intellectual activities such as depicting the experience through art or writing. More often, the adolescent will want to gain a sense of mastery by talking about the experience. The preparator should be available to the adolescent for this. The preparator can also introduce other adolescents who have had similar, or at least other health care experiences. The adolescents' peer support can enhance mastery in one another.

The adolescent has a further need that is not so evident in younger children. This is his need to know the results of the procedure. Because the adolescent is able to consider the possible outcomes of the procedure and their implications in his life, he will be anxious to know the results of the procedure. The results can be discussed with the adolescent and he can be told what can be expected to happen next. This information must be accurately based on the physician's plans. The preparator might arrange this discussion between tbe adolescent and physician. This understanding lays the gound work for the adolescent's mastery-in-advance for whatever might be ahead for him.

SUMMARY

Preparation for diagnostic procedures has been discussed in each of five age groupings. These groupings are based on the development of abilities as derived from the theories of Piaget and Erikson. Cognitive and psychosocial developmental implications on the process of preparation have been discussed in relation to the child's development of trust, understanding, and mastery of the diagnostic procedure. Environmental and individual influences on the child's preparation must be considered, since the developmental knowledge provides the base for planning the child's preparation.

The family can help the child cope with health care events such as diagnostic procedures. The parents' anxiety is reflected in the child's anxiety. For these reasons, the parents should be prepared and should be included in the child's preparation wherever possible.

The preparator must become acquainted with the child and the family and must learn how developmental, environmental, and personal influences affect the child's ability to cope. This assessment forms the basis for the establishment of a therapeutic alliance with the child, the presentation of preparation information, the choice of which concrete experiences to include, and for the plan for the child's mastery of the experience.

When the preparator has facilitated the child's trust, understanding, and mastery, the process of preparation has taken place. This process has been found to decrease and make manageable the child's fears and anxieties aroused by diagnostic procedures. Thus, the preparator has played a significant role in helping the child cope, and enhancing the child's ability to deal with future stressful experiences.

REFERENCE

1. Erikson E: *Childhood and Society*. New York, Norton, 1950.

BIBLIOGRAPHY

Becker RO: Therapeutic approaches to psychopathological reactions to hospitalization. *Int J Child Psychother* 1(2):65, 1972.

Ditman LL: A child's sense of trust. *Am J Nurs* 66(1):91, 1966.

Erickson F: Play interviews for four-year-old hospitalized children. *Monogr Soc Res Child Dev* 23:1, 1958.

Freud A: The role of bodily illness in the mental life of children. *Psychoanalytic study of the child* 7:69, 1952.

Gellert E (ed): *Psychosocial aspects of pediatric care.* New York, Grune and Stratton, 1978.

Johnson JE, Kirschkoff KT, Eddress MP: Easing children's fright during health care procedures. *Matern Child Nurs J* 1(July-Aug):206, 1976.

Knight RB, Atkins A, Eagle CJ, et al;: Psychological stress, ego defenses and cortisol production in children hospitalized for elective surgery. *Psychosom. Med* 42(1):40, 1979.

Levy DM: Psychic trauma of operations in children. *Am J Dis Child* 69:7, 1945.

Maier HW: *Three theories of child development.* New York, Harper and Row, Publishers, Inc, 1969.

Melamed BG, Meyer R, Gei C, et al: The influence of time and type of preparation on children's adjustment to hospitalization. *J Pediatr Psychol* 1(4):31–37, 1976.

Melamed BG, Siegel LJ: Reduction of anxiety in children facing hospitalization and surgery by use of filmed modeling. *J Consult Clin Psychol* 43(4):511, 1975.

Murphy LB, Moriarity AE: *Vulnerability, Coping, and Growth.* New Haven, Yale University Press, 1976.

Petrillo M, Sanger S: *Emotional care of hospitalized children.* Philadelphia, JB Lippincott Co, 1972.

Piaget J: *The language and thought of the child.* New York, Meridian Books, 1955.

Plank E: *Working with children in hospitals,* ed. 2. Cleveland, Ohio, Case-Western Reserve University Press, 1971.

Prugh DG, Staub EM, Sands HH, Kirschbaum RM, Lenihan EA: A study of the emotional reactions of children and families to hospitalization and illness. *Am J Orthopsychiatry* 23:70–106, 1953.

Robertson J: *Young children in hospitals.* New York, Basic Books, 1958.

Schrader E: Preparation play helps children in hospitals. *AORN J* 30(2):336, 1979.

Siegel LJ: Preparation of children for hospitalization: a selected review of the research literature. *J Pediatr Psychol* 1(4):26–30, 1976.

Skipper J, Leonard R: Children, stress, and hospitalization: a field experiment. *J Health Soc Behav* 9:275–287, 1968.

Vernon DT, Bailey WC: The use of motion pictures in the psychological preparation of children for induction of anesthesia. *Anesthesiology* 40:68, 1974.

Vernon DTA, Foley JM, Sipowicz RR, et al: *The psychological responses of children to hospitalization and illness.* Springfield, Ill, Charles C Thomas Publisher, 1965.

Visintainer M, Wolfer JA: Psychological preparation for surgical pediatric patients: the effects on children's and parents' stress responses and adjustment. *Pediatrics* 56:187, 1975.

Watson J: Research and literature on children's response to injections: some general nursing implications. *Pediatr Nurs* 2(1):7–8, 1976.

Wu R: Explaining treatments to young children. *Am J Nurs* 65(7):71, 1965.

3

The Child's Consent to Treatment

Linda C. Hoot

It is imperative that the health practitioner understand the child's rights if she is to function within the legal framework of professional practice. A growing concern within the various health care systems becomes apparent when determining a child's right to consent to treatment. As more and more young people begin to live apart from the family, there are larger numbers of minors seeking health care independently of their parents. Concomitant with these increasing numbers, there is the need to understand the laws applicable to the practioner, child, and parent. A conflict arises when the desires of the minor go against those of the parent. The question of treatment is most critical when dealing with young people between the ages of 13 and 16 years. A minor's eligibility to give consent to treatment is based on his age, freedom from parental control, intelligence, general conduct as an adult, economic status, employment, and training (1). Determination of majority varies from state to state; therefore, it is advisable that the health practitioner become familiar with the individual guidelines established by the state in which he or she intends to practice. The following pages stress that the child's developmental status should be considered when determining his right to give consent for treatment. For the purpose of this discussion, the rights of the child to informed consent refers to the rights of the parent or guardian, acting as the child's advocate, to informed consent. In addition, the practitioner should be aware of the wishes of the maturing adolescent.

The purposes of this chapter are fourfold:

- to identify the legal rights of the child as related to a diagnostic procedure

- to list the responsibilities of the child's parents or guardian as the advocate of the child's rights
- to describe the nurse's role in safeguarding the rights of the child
- to state the rights of the parent or guardian of the child

In order to function within the legal framework of nursing, the health care provider must fully understand her role in obtaining consent to treatment.

RIGHTS IN HEALTH CARE

In the delivery of health care, it has been established that each person has certain rights. By definition, a right is a privilege secured by law, which must not be violated unless specific consent is given. When the health care provider does not meet the standards established by the medical community, the term *malpractice* is used. The law provides that all people have a right to full disclosure as they seek health care. In the context of the health professions, disclosure can be defined as providing the client with adequate information so that he is able to weigh the pros and cons of a situation in order to decide on a therapeutic course of action.

In the absence of an emergency, parental consent must be obtained before a child is treated. Such consent is mandatory since children are considered fundamentally incapable of giving consent (2). Therefore, it becomes the responsibility of the health practitioner to provide the parent with information regarding the care and treatment to be rendered. The information provided to the parent about the child should be based on the same standards of informed consent as afforded to an adult.

Parents as well as society play valuable roles as the child's advocate, thereby insuring quality medical treatment. The remainder of this chapter will be dedicated to providing the health practioner with the knowledge necessary for her to obtain informed consent in the treatment of the child.

DISCLOSURE AS A MECHANISM FOR INFORMED CONSENT

Paramount in the mind of the health practitioner should be the question, "What information should be given to the parent in order to have informed consent?" In answering this question, it is mandatory that the nurse realize that the nurse-client relationship is a fiduciary relationship, one based on trust and confidence. In this type of relationship, one person is considered to be an expert in the field and the other person is considered to be less knowledgeable. It is the responsibility of the expert to fully disclose to the novice the details of the situation.

Disclosure is a prerequisite for valid consent. When informing the parent, it has been suggested that the standards for disclosure established by the Federal Drug Administration be used as guidelines when procuring consent to treatment (3). These guidelines include:

1. Diagnosis of the illness
2. Nature of the treatment
3. Purpose of the treatment and expected duration
4. Methods used to administer the treatment
5. Discussion of any risks or hazards involved (including possible side effects)
6. Alternative forms of treatment
7. Benefits that are expected of the treatment
8. Prognosis should the parent refuse the treatment

When disclosing the necessary information to the parents, the health practitioner must be warned to avoid
"filling in the gaps." Should an omission in the parent's
knowledge be noticed by the nurse, she should discuss this
omission with the physician before mentioning it to the
parent. The nurse should avoid over- and underdisclosure.
Overdisclosure may lead to undue anxiety in the parent,
whereas underdisclosure may be interpreted as deception.

Disclosure is a complex issue. It is often difficult for the
health practitioner to determine exactly what is sufficient
information for the parent to make an informed consent.
When assessing the parent's right to know, the practitioner
who exhibits honest concern for her patient will have most
success in obtaining informed consent.

THE NURSE'S RESPONSIBILITY AND INFORMED CONSENT

Any clerk in the hospital can have parents sign a consent
form. It is not necessary that the professional nurse be
present at the signing of the consent form. It is the
physician's, not the nurse's, responsibility to provide a
parent or guardian with explanations of impending medical and/or surgical treatment. This responsibility cannot
be delegated to the nurse.

Although the professional nurse is not legally responsible for explaining the impending procedure(s), she still
has an important responsibility in the area of informed
consent. The professional nurse's role is twofold in this
area:

1. Education
2. Evaluation

Education

The professional nurse has a distinct role in patient education. In providing everyday nursing care, the nurse is constantly requesting permission from the patient to invade his environment. This request may be in the form of either a verbal or written request. Each time the nurse invades the patient's environment, she must, either formally or informally, request his permission to do so. In making this request, the nurse who informs her patient of the rationale for the invasion is more likely to receive his permission than the nurse who simply requests permission without explanation. For example, as the nurse prepares a patient for a diagnostic procedure, she must make certain requests of that patient. It remains the prerogative of the patient, in this case, the parent, to deny permission. If the nurse explains the need for the preparation in a nonthreatening manner, the request may be more easily granted. In the event the request is denied, the nurse's only alternative is to respect the parent's or guardian's wish and report the situation to the physician.

Evaluation

As stated previously, the professional nurse does not necessarily have to be present when a consent form is signed. This is a duty that can be delegated by the physician to any number of people. It is, however, the duty of the health professional to evaluate whether or not the person giving consent is fully aware of all possible consequences of the procedure. If consent is obtained when full disclosure has not been provided by the physician, the consent is not valid.

As the nurse evaluates the parent's understanding of the procedure, she should keep in mind the following: is the parent (1) conscious and aware of what is being signed, (2) informed regarding the nature, as well as the calculated risks, and (3) ready and willing to execute the consent voluntarily and without duress? Should the nurse find that the parent is in any of the above ways uninformed, the consent form should not be signed. The nurse should immediately inform the appropriate person so that the physician can be notified, a solution can be found, and truly informed consent can be obtained (4).

THE CONSENT FORM

As stated earlier, the consent form should be filled out only after the physician has fully explained to the child's parent or guardian what the procedure is and all possible risks of the procedure. Guidelines established by the Health Law Center (5) suggest that a consent form be obtained whenever any of the following are anticipated:

1. Anesthesia
2. Major or minor surgery
3. Procedures that could involve harm to the patient, for example, pyelography and angiography
4. Cobalt or x-ray therapy
5. Electroshock therapy
6. Experimental procedures
7. Any other procedure for which the medical staff deems consent to be necessary.

When in doubt as to the need for written consent, consent should be obtained.

For the purposes of clarification, a case study has been developed to help the practitioner understand how to complete a consent form.

Case Study: Janice H. Lee, a 5-year-old girl, is admitted to the hospital by Dr. Susan L. Augusta. The admitting diagnosis is glomerulonephritis. During the course of Janice's stay in the hospital, Dr. Augusta elects to perform a renal biopsy.

Figure 3-1 is an example of one type of completed special procedure consent form.

Important points to remember when completing all consent forms include:

1. Use the terminology of lay people.
2. Avoid abbreviations except in the case of a middle initial.
3. Fill in all blanks before obtaining the patient's or parent's signature.
4. Fill in the exact time the consent form was signed.
5. Witnesses should be 18 years of age or older.

TREATMENT OF A CHILD WHEN THE PARENT REFUSES

When a diagnostic procedure for a child is being considered, the parent's or guardian's wish must be respected. The only recourse a practitioner has in obtaining consent to treatment when the parent or guardian refuses is through the legal action of declaring negligence on the part of the parent or guardian. When a condition is a threat to the life and/or well-being of the child, the parent's right to custody can be removed by the court so that the child can be treated. In addition to a life-threatening situation, the risks to the child's biological, psychological, and social development must be considered. The child's

Figure 3-1

Special procedure consent form.

Patient _____ Age _____

                                                              AM
Date _____ Time _____ PM

1. I, _____ (patient), do hereby give my
                                                authorization

   to Dr. _____ and/or the physician
                                                designated, to perform
   the following special procedure, examination, or treatment:

   _____

   _____

   _____

   (A description of the procedure(s) in language of laymen)

2. I also authorize the attending physician, and/or designated
   physician, to perform the above procedure, examination or
   treatment, to do any other procedure that, in the judgment of
   the physician, may be advisable on the above patient.

3. The nature and purpose of the procedure, treatment, or
   examination, risks involved, and the possibility of
   complications have been explained to me. These are:

   _____

   _____

   _____

4. I also understand that there are further risks involved in this
   procedure that are risks involved in the performance of any

60

surgical procedure. They may include cardiac arrest, respiratory arrest, death, severe blood loss, etc. It is my understanding that no guarantees have been provided to me as a result of consenting to this procedure.

5. I consent to the administration of anesthetics to be applied by or under the direction and supervision of

Dr. _____, and to the use of such anesthetics as he may deem advisable in my case.

6. I certify that I have read and fully understand the above consent, that the explanations referred to were made, and that all blanks or statements requiring insertion or completion were filled in before I affixed my signature.

_____

(Patient's signature)

_____

(Witness)

_____

(Witness)

If patient is a minor or unable to sign, complete the following:

Patient is a minor, _____
years of age, or is unable to sign, because _____

_____

_____   _____
(Father)   (Guardian)

_____   _____
(Mother)   (Guardian)

_____

61

wishes should also be evaluated. As the practitioner and/
or court weighs the variables identified above, the potential
risks and benefits of the procedure must be considered.
When the courts decide in the favor of the parent, charges
of battery can be brought against the practitioner should
treatment be instituted against parental desires (6).

INFORMED CONSENT IN AN EMERGENCY

Consent to treat a child must be obtained from a parent
or guardian except in the presence of an emergency. In
the absence of the parent or guardian, consent may be
obtained from other sources. Each state has defined those
people who are authorized to give consent in the absence
of the parent or guardian. An emergency is any situation
that threatens the immediate life and/or well-being of the
patient. However, it behooves the practitioner to understand that the legal definition of emergency may vary
from state to state. In an emergency situation, when
treatment is provided and consent is not obtained, the
practitioner should be able to prove, through documen-
tation, that consent could not be obtained and treatment
was necessary in order to maintain the well-being of the
patient.

Although a suit can be filed against the health care
provider when emergency treatment is provided without
consent, the practitioner who thoroughly documents the
circumstances surrounding the action taken is better able
to prove the need for the emergency treatment and
therefore be supported in a legal case.

SUMMARY

To summarize, it is imperative that the nurse understand
the rights of all individuals. Informed consent imposes
legal constraint on health care providers as individuals

and on the institutions in a variety of settings. If the nurse is to function within a legal framework, she must understand the full impact of patient consent.

REFERENCES

1. Holder AR: *Legal Issues in Pediatrics and Adolescent Medicine.* New York, John Wiley & Sons, 1977, p 135.
2. Holder AR: *Legal Issues in Pediatrics and Adolescent Medicine.* New York, John Wiley & Sons, 1977, p 148.
3. "Informed Consent—A Proposed Standard for Medical Disclosure." *New York University Law Review.* 48(3):555–557, 1973.
4. Regan WA: "Nurses and Surgical Consent Forms." *Regan Report on Nursing Law,* December 1973, p 1.
5. *Problems in Hospital Law,* ed 2. Rockville, Maryland, Aspen Corporation, 1974, p 79.
6. *Problems in Hospital Law,* ed 2. Rockville, Maryland, Aspen Corporation, 1974, p 85.

BIBLIOGRAPHY

Alton WG: *Malpractice: A Trial Lawyer's Advice for Physicians (How to Avoid, How to Win).* Boston, Little, Brown & Co, 1977.

Annas GJ: *The Rights of Hospital Patients.* New York, Avon Books, 1975.

Creighton H: *Law Every Nurse Should Know,* ed 3. Philadelphia, WB Saunders Co, 1975.

Holder AR: *Legal Issues in Pediatrics and Adolescent Medicine.* New York, John Wiley & Sons, 1977.

"Informed Consent—A Proposed Standard for Medical Disclosure." *New York University Law Review,* 48(3):548–563, 1973.

Katz J: *Experimentation with Human Beings.* New York, Russell Sage Foundation, 1972.

Maritz AR, Morris RC: *Handbook of Legal Medicine.* St Louis, CV Mosby Co, 1975.

Murchison I, Nichols TS, Hanson R: *Legal Accountability in the Nursing Process.* St Louis, CV Mosby Co, 1978.

Nursing and the Law, ed 2. The Health Law Center, Streiff CJ, Esq, (eds). Rockville, Maryland, Aspen Corporation, 1975.

Problem in Hospital Law, ed 2. Rockville, Maryland, Aspen Corporation, 1974.

Regan, WA: "Nurses and Surgical Consent Forms." *Regan Report on Nursing Law* 8:14, 1973.

Rothman DA, Rothman NL: "The Nurse and Informed Consent." *J Nurs Adm* 12(3):7–9, 1977.

Sorensen KC, Luckmann J: *Basic Nursing: A Psychophysiologic Approach.* Philadelphia, WB Saunders Co, 1979.

Willy SH: *The Nurse's Guide to the Law.* New York, McGraw-Hill Book Co, 1970.

4

Cardiovascular Diagnostic Procedures

BONE MARROW ASPIRATION

Bone marrow aspiration is an invasive procedure used to diagnose a wide variety of hematologic disorders. Peripheral blood studies, which are done first, give an indication of the diagnosis.

Premedication: None.

Diet: No restriction necessary.

Consent: An authorization signed by the parent or guardian is necessary.

Time: 10 minutes.

Procedure: Various sites are used to obtain a specimen of bone marrow; the most common sites are the posterior and anterior iliac crests and the proximal end of the tibia. The tibiae are not used as sites after 18 months of age because of increased thickness of bone cortex. For older children, the spinous processes of the vertebrae, or ribs may also be used. The sternum is seldom used in children because of increased risk of perforation to the mediastinum. If repeated aspirations or biopsy specimens are needed, several sites may be used.

   Positioning of the patient depends on the area to be punctured:

1. When the anterior iliac crests are used, the patient lies flat on his back.
2. If marrow is to be aspirated from the tibia, the child can be restrained most easily on his back or side.
3. When the vertebral spinous processes are used, the patient sits up and leans forward, or may be placed on his abdomen with a firm support under his hips to provide flexion of the back.
4. When the posterior ilium is the site of choice, the patient lies on his side, head flexed onto chest, and knees drawn up to the abdomen. The nurse or assistant plays an important role in helping the child remain immobile in these positions.

After the patient is positioned, the skin is cleansed with a disinfectant solution and sterile towels are draped around the site. Then the skin, subcutaneous tissues, and periosteum are infiltrated with a local anesthetic.

The nurse can offer distraction and support while the anesthetic is taking effect. When the area is anesthetized, the clinician inserts an 18 gauge marrow needle through the cortex to the bone with a slight twisting motion. Then the stylet is removed, the hub of the needle is attached to a 10 ml syringe, and 0.2–0.5 ml of fluid is aspirated. The needle is removed and pressure is applied at the puncture site for a few minutes with a 4 × 4 sterile gauze.

Preparation: The child should be prepared for the following: the removal of clothing, usually pants if the iliac crest is used; a cold sensation as the skin is cleansed with a disinfectant; the positioning of sterile towels around the site; a stinging or burning sensation as local anesthetic is injected into the subcutaneous tissues and periosteum; a feeling of pressure as a needle is inserted through the cortex of the bone; moderately severe pain of a few seconds duration as suction is applied to the needle; removal of the needle as soon as the bone marrow has been aspirated; and pressure at the puncture site for a few minutes with a sterile 4 × 4 gauze.

Restraint Necessary: The child will need to be restrained securely from the time he is positioned until the needle is removed. This can be accomplished effectively in a number of ways, depending on the site of the aspiration.

If the posterior ilium site is used, the nurse places one hand behind the child's neck and the other under his buttocks. By resting her body gently on the child's body and by applying pressure on the neck and legs, she can round his back and keep it parallel to the side of the table. If the child must be in a supine position, a "mummy board" is useful. When such a device is not available, at least two people are needed to help the child remain immobile during the procedure.

As is always the case with restraint, the child must be given a clear explanation of the purpose and duration of the restraint. (See Appendix A, "Restraining Infants and Children.")

Aftercare: The patient should be observed for bleeding from the site, discomfort, or any other untoward symptoms. If the procedure is performed on an outpatient basis, the child should remain on the premises for approximately 30 minutes for observation.

Interpretation of Findings: The specimen should be sent immediately to the hematology laboratory for staining and evaluation. This evaluation will include marrow cellularity; types of cells present, including presence or absence of cells foreign to the marrow; maturation of the cellular marrow elements; and composition and extent of supporting marrow connective tissue. (See Appendix B for normal values.)

CARDIAC CATHETERIZATION

Paula Dimmitt

Cardiac catheterization is an invasive procedure in which a catheter (a thin hollow tube) is inserted into an arm or leg vessel and passed to the heart. The purpose of this procedure is to obtain cardiac blood samples, pressures, and to facilitate injection of a dye into preselected parts of the heart (Fig. 4-1). This procedure helps to diagnose and clarify congenital heart disease for proper medical or surgical treatment. Also, it provides an evaluation of postoperative cardiac repair.

The preparation, procedure, and aftercare for peripheral, thoracic, or abdominal angiograms are the same. The normal values would depend on the disease entity.

Premedication: Generally a mixture of a narcotic or a barbiturate and a sedative to produce a relaxed, sleepy child is administered intramuscularly approximately 30 minutes to an hour before the scheduled catheterization. These are a few of the suggested combinations:

1. Morphine and pentobarbital
2. Droperidol and meperidine
3. Morphine, pentobarbital, and chlorpromazine
4. Meperidine, promethazine, and chlorpromazine

It is not a general practice to premedicate newborns and infants weighing 5 kilograms or less.

Diet: The precatheterization diet for an infant still receiving feedings between 11 PM and 7 AM is not interrupted until 4 hours before the scheduled procedure. At that time, the infant cannot be fed any liquids or food until after the procedure. Older children are kept without food or liquids after midnight before the morning of the procedure.

The postcatheterization diet for all ages starts with clear liquids. It then progresses to a full regular diet after the effects of the premedication subside.

Consent: A formal, informed operative permit, signed by the parents or a legal guardian, is required by most states and hospitals.

Time: A cardiac catheterization may be as short as 30 minutes or as long as 3 hours.

Procedure: Xylocaine is infiltrated into the chosen site. The choice of site depends on what the physician wants to accomplish.

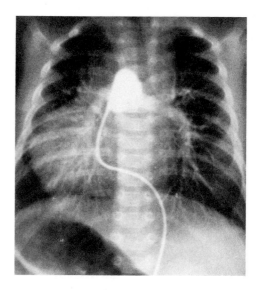

Figure 4-1
X-ray film taken during a cardiac catheterization. Dye has been injected into the pulmonary artery.

A right heart catheterization is feasible through a venous entry. The preferred venous entries are the saphenous vein in the groin or the basilic vein in the arm. The saphenous vein can be entered by performing a cutdown or by a percutaneous entry. A percutaneous entry is similar to starting an IV, a long needle is inserted to make a hole in the skin and into the vessel. Through this hole, a catheter is inserted. The percutaneous method can be employed in the groin only. The cutdown method may be used in the arm or groin. The method of entry chosen depends on the physician's preference.

The left side of the heart can be entered from the right side of the heart through a formamen ovale, an atrial, or a ventricular septal defect. If this is not possible, a left heart catheterization can be accomplished through a cutdown or percutaneous entry of the femoral artery in the groin or a cutdown on the brachial artery in the arm.

Once the catheter is inserted into the chosen vessel, its course up to and inside the heart is visualized on the fluorscopy screen. The catheter is manipulated by the cardiologist through each area of the internal heart and its vessels.

The following data are obtained in each area:

1. Intracardiac pressures are recorded on light-sensitive paper for a permanent record.
2. Oxygen saturations are obtained to check for possible desaturation of the blood in the heart.
3. Blood gases may be obtained to further delineate any desaturation.
4. Radiopaque dye is injected into selected chambers and vessels of the heart. The dye mixes with the blood and makes it appear black on the fluorscopy screen, thus outlining the heart and vessels. This is recorded on video tape and an actual movie film is made for a permanent record.

After this information is obtained, the catheter is removed and the cutdown vein ligated (tied off with suture) and the skin sutured. A cutdown on the arterial vessel would generally require repair of the artery and overlying skin with sutures.

A percutaneous entry in either kind of vessel only requires manual pressure over the entry site to help form a clot at the site.

A dressing may consist of an antibiotic ointment at the entry site covered by a Band-Aid or pressure dressing.

Preparation: The physical preparation is divided into two areas, medical and nursing.

The medical preparation consists of:

1. Physical examination by a pediatric cardiologist.
2. Electrocardiogram (EKG or ECG)
3. Chest roentgerogram: posterior/anterior (PA) and lateral views.
4. Echocardiogram
5. Complete blood count (CBC)

The nursing preparation consists of:

1. Measurement of vital signs: pulse, temperature, respirations, and blood pressure every eight hours.
2. No liquids or foods (NPO) after a designated time set according to the child's age. To prevent accidental ingestion of liquids or foods, attach an NPO sign to the bed or the patient, if necessary. Also, remove all liquids and foods from the bedside.
3. Have the child change into hospital pajamas. Request that children not wear any underclothing so it does not get misplaced and lost when removed for the catheterization.
4. Have the child void (urinate) just before administering the premedication. The dye injection causes the kidneys to filtrate rapidly and fill up the bladder quickly. Voiding before the sedative injection avoids the chance of the child falling while going to the bathroom.

5. Remove any nail polish from the fingernails and toenails. This allows easy assessment of peripheral cyanosis at any time.
6. Remove glasses, jewelry, or body braces.
7. Check that the proper identification band is in place on the child.
8. Give the premedication when ordered.

Record all the above information on the chart in the nurses' notes and check off each step of the preoperative checklist. Fill in the requested information on the Cardiac Catheterization Nursing Record under Pre-Cath Visit (Fig. 4-2).

The psychological preparation is necessary for many reasons. In order to reduce the child's and the parents' fears and anxieties, information should be presented at the time of admission. This provides them with the opportunity to anticipate and understand each event.

The teaching must be simple and truthful so that the child's sense of trust can be maintained and the parents can provide appropriate emotional support throughout the hospitalization.

The long-range goal of this preparation is to prevent any lasting emotional trauma. This is accomplished by playing with the child and using terms for his age level. The major points of the information are:

1. Admitting procedure.
   a. Finger stick "blood test" (some children call it a shot).
   b. Urination into a cup: "Potty into a little cup."
   c. Blood pressure, temperature, pulse, and name band.
2. Reason for coming to the hospital.*

---

*Using a stethoscope to let the child or teenager hear his own heart helps him to identify the heart and where it is located. The teenager or older child may benefit from looking at a diagram of the heart and seeing where the defect is located.

Small child: "The doctor heard an extra (or different) sound in your heart and wants to take a picture of your heart."

Teenager: "The doctor hears a murmur, which means (name the defect and explain it). This means that the

CHILDREN'S MEDICAL CENTER
OF DALLAS

CARDIAC CATHETERIZATION   Date:
NURSING RECORD   Time:

PRE-CATH VISIT

Preferred Name: _____

Allergies: No _____ Yes _____

Special Medications or IV's: No _____ Yes _____

Blood: No _____ Yes _____ Product & Quantity _____

Anesthesia: No _____ Yes _____ Anesthesia Staff: _____ Anesthesia Resident: _____

Prosthesis: No _____ Glasses: _____ Hearing Aid: _____ Other: _____

Skin: Nothing Abnormal _____ Cyanotic _____ Rash _____ Bruises _____ Bites _____

Location on Body: _____

Language Spoken: English _____ Spanish _____ Other: _____

Feed: Bottle _____ Breast _____ Cup _____

Toilet Trained: No _____ Yes _____

Specific requests of patient and/or parents: _____

Assessment and Teaching: _____

Dopler B/P: (R) Arm _____ (L) Arm _____ ; (R) Leg: D.P. _____ P.T. _____ ; (L) Leg: D.P. _____ P.T. _____

Pulses: _____ Capillary Filling: Good _____ Fair _____ Absent _____

Skin Temp: Warm _____ Cool _____   Color: Normal _____ Abnormal _____

POST-CATH VISIT   Date: _____   Time: _____

Cath Site: Nothing Abnormal _____ Bruised _____ Reddened _____ Swollen _____ Rash_____

Assessment and Teaching: _____

Dopler B/P: (R) Arm _____ (L) Arm _____ ; (R) Leg: D.P. _____ P.T. _____ ; (L) Leg: D.P. _____ P.T. _____

Pulses: _____ Capillary Filling: Good _____ Fair _____ Absent _____

Skin Temp: Warm _____ Cool _____   Color: Normal _____ Abnormal _____

Figure 4-2

Cardiac catheterization nursing record. (Courtesy of Children's Medical Center, Dallas, Texas.) (Figure continued on pages 76-77.)

CHILDREN'S MEDICAL CENTER
OF DALLAS

CARDIAC CATHETERIZATION NURSING RECORD

	Weight Kg	Height cm	Hemoglobin	Hematocrit	Admission Pulse	Admission Resp.	Admission B/P
TIME							/
Rectal Temp. C°							
Pulse							
Resp.							
B/P Syst. / Dyst.							
Valium IV							
Heparin IV							
Protamine Sulfate IV							
O₂ %							
Activity							
Resp.							
Circ.							
Conscious							
Color							

SCORING GUIDE

Activity
2 = moves purposefully
1 = moves involuntarily
0 = not moving

Respiration
2 = regular Resp. - coughs/cries
1 = distressed or periodic
0 = requires ventilation

Circulation
2 = +/− 20% pre-op systolic BP
1 = +/− 20-50% pre-op BP
0 = +/− 50% or more pre-op BP
* = arrythmia - lower score 1 point

Consciousness
2 = awake
1 = arousable
0 = not responding

Color
2 = pink
1 = abnormal color/appearance
0 = cyanotic

PRE-OP MEDS:

	Time	Observations
		Arrived in Cath Lab

Intake

FLUIDS HUNG IN CATH LAB

	Total cc	Metriset	
☐ D5RL			cc
☐ D5W			cc
☐ D4MRL			cc
☐			cc
☐ BLOOD			cc

FLUIDS FROM FLOOR

	Total cc	Metriset	
☐ D5RL			cc
☐ D5W			cc
☐ D4MRL			cc

Flush D_5 in 0.2% NaCl — cc
Dye — Reno — M — 60 — cc
P.O. — D_5W — cc
TOTAL RECEIVED =

OUTPUT

Blood (estimated) — cc
Urine (estimated) — cc
Vomitus (estimated) — cc
BM (estimated) — cc

	YES	NO
Blood Type Drawn — Sent to Lab		
T & C Drawn — Sent to Lab		
KUB Taken		
Dopler B/P Study		

CATH SITE

PERCUTANEOUS:
Vein: ® Leg ☐ Leg ☐
Artery: ® Leg ☐ Leg ☐

CUTDOWN:
Lig'd. Rep'd.
Vein: ® ☐ ☐
Artery: ® ☐ ☐

DRESSING

Betadine Oint. ☐
Bandaid ☐
Pressure ☐
Collodion ☐

COMPLICATIONS

None ☐
Bleeding ☐
Elev. Temp. ☐
Dye Reaction ☐
Bradycardia ☐
Tachycardia ☐
Block ☐
Resp. Arrest ☐
Cardiac Arrest ☐

EKG LEADS #
R   L

Cardiologist _____

R.N. _____

Anesthesiologist: _____

SCORE ENTERING CATH LAB
1 - 2 - 3 - 4 - 5 - 6 - 7 - 8 - 9 - 10
SCORE LEAVING CATH LAB
1 - 2 - 3 - 4 - 5 - 6 - 7 - 8 - 9 - 10

Figure 4-2 (Continued)

doctor needs to take a picture of the inside of your heart."

3. Hospital room appearance.

4. Playroom or other recreational facilities.

5. Eating and sleeping at the hospital with a parent.

6. Activities of catheterization morning:

　　a. Change into hospital pajamas: "No underpants or shorts. You will have to take the pajamas off for the pictures, and we don't want to lose your pajamas or undershorts." Emphasize that a sheet will cover him, so that the child or teenager does not think he will be lying there exposed.

　　b. No breakfast or liquids: "Empty your tummy."
　　　　Small child: "We do not want to take a picture of your food, just of your heart."
　　　　Teenager: "The dye injection (liquid medicine that helps the doctor see the inside structures of your heart) can upset your stomach if you've eaten."

　　c. "OK to brush your teeth."

　　d. Importance of urination: "Empty bladder to decrease the urge during the catheterization."
　　　　Teenager: Clarify that this urge is strongest during the dye injection.

　　e. Premedication injection "to make you sleepy."
　　　　Injection Receiving Technique:
　　　　(1) Tell the child to lay on his back with his legs straight (promotes self-control).
　　　　(2) Tell him to hold hands with his parents (for security and restraint).
　　　　(3) Tell him to look at his parents. "Keep your eyes wide open" (promotes reality and thus conscious control).
　　　　(4) Tell him to yell "ouch" when the injection hurts. (release of tension).
　　　　(5) Have the young child and his parents count until the end of the injection (shows child how short the shot is and gives him and his parents something

to do during the injection). Have the teenager count while visualizing numbers in the air (creates mind-over-body control and promotes muscle relaxation; demonstrate muscle tightness and show how hard a muscle can be by flexing the arm muscle).

(6) Place a Band-Aid on the injection site (makes it feel better and is a badge of courage for a young child, especially with a picture drawn on it).

(7) Rub his leg hard or bicycle his legs while the child is lying down (releases tension through physical activity, promotes circulation of medication, and decreases muscle soreness).

(8) Tell the child to stay in bed after the injection: "I don't want you to fall asleep on the floor after your shot."

f. Transportation to the catheterization lab: Parents are to say "see you later" in the room and not accompany the child to the laboratory. This emphasizes "see you later" and allows time for the nurse and child to continue the relationship begun in the previous days' teaching.

7. Procedure: Mention only what can be seen, heard, and felt by the child.

   a. Pajamas are removed and body is covered by a sheet.

   b. Arms are restrained above his head snugly (demonstrate by putting his arms up and explain that the arms would get in the way when taking pictures of the heart).

   c. Legs are restrained far apart, knees point to the outside.

   d. ECG leads attached to all four limbs, called *buttons* for a small child.

   e. Caps and masks should be worn by everyone except the child. "The doctor and nurses cover their hair and nose and mouth. You can still see their eyes, though."

f. Groin or arm area is washed. Emphasize this is the only time they are uncovered.

g. Shot to "put the skin to sleep." Use *Injection Receiving Technique.*

h. Lights are dimmed for the "movie picture." A younger child is told to nap so he can remain very still for the picture, and emphasize that there will be no more shots.
   A teenager is told to stay very still and can watch the "television" (fluoscopy screen).

i. Describe the angiogram to the older child and teen-ager.
   (1) Loud movie camera sound.
   (2) Warm or hot feeling all over for 15 seconds.
   (3) Odd taste in mouth.
   (4) Urge to urinate.
   (5) Tell him to breathe slowly in and out of mouth during this time.

j. Dressing or Band-Aid applied.
   Younger child: "over injection area."
   Teenager: "over catheter insertion site." The teen-ager and his parents are shown a small catheter and shown how it is manipulated.

k. The child is transferred to his own room or the recovery room ("wake-up room" for the younger child who takes a nap).

8. He is instructed to keep bandaged leg or arm straight. He may have clear soda and is not allowed out of bed until the designated time. The use of a bedpan or urinal is explained:
   Younger child: "Bed potty or bottle."

The emotional response of the child and parents should be recorded on the Cardiac Catheterization Nursing Record under the section "Assessment and Teaching" (Fig. 4-3).

An important trend is developing in the psychological preparation of children for this and other procedures.

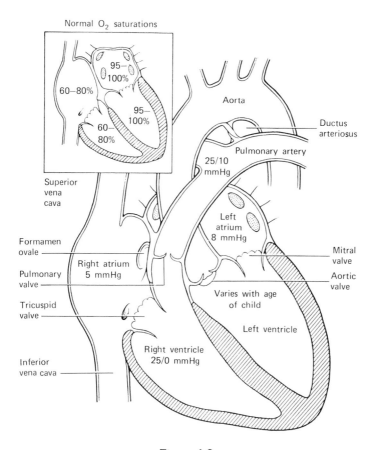

Figure 4-3

Normal intracardiac pressures. (Courtesy of Alvis F. Johnson, Jr., MD, Children's Medical Center, Dallas, Texas.)

Various teaching aids have been developed that may be given to the child and his parents before they come to the hospital. These teaching aids are to be used at home. For example, coloring books with pictures of the hospital and catheterization events, and simple, age level explanations are good teaching aids. This promotes communication between parent and the child in the safe, familiar home environment by familiarizing the family with the upcoming hospital events. Teaching is best started at home by the people the child trusts most, the parents.

Aftercare: The two main objectives of nursing aftercare are the prevention of nausea and vomiting and of potential hemorrhage at the catheterized site. Also, the nurse needs to anticipate and evaluate the potential formation of a clot blocking a blood vessel, cardiac arrhythmias, and cyanotic episodes.

When the child returns from the cardiac catheterization, bedrest and immobilization of the catheterized limb are necessary. The amount of both depends on the method and site of catheterization. The information about the method and site can be obtained from the Intracardiac Catheterization Nursing Record (Fig. 4-3).

If the cutdown method is used, the child is usually allowed up for bathroom privileges by evening. A percutaneous method usually requires that the child be at complete bedrest until the next morning.

If bleeding should occur at the catheterized site, apply manual pressure for 10 minutes and a new dressing. Report the occurrence in the nurses' notes and advise the cardiologist.

Immobilization requires that the catheterized limb be kept straight and still until the above-mentioned time periods have elapsed. Generally, the child will voluntarily keep the limb straight and still, especially if instructed to do this before and after the catheterization. Constant reinforcement by the parents is also helpful. If the femoral area was percutaneously entered, sitting upright in bed is not permitted since this bends the femoral vessels. When placing the child on a bedpan, apply pressure to the dressing when lifting on and off. This helps prevent site bleeding. Apply pressure at the site if the child should vomit. The abdominal strain that occurs while vomiting frequently causes bleeding at the catheterized site. This is particularly true in the older or teenaged child.

The vital signs and blood pressure should be compared

to the intracardiac and postcardiac catheterization readings. The vital signs and blood pressure should be taken at least every hour for 4 hours. Also, the pulses, color, warmth, and capillary filling of the catheterized limb should be checked and charted every hour for 4 hours. The following charting of pulses is recommended:

0: Pulse is not palpable.

+1: Pulse is thready, weak, and difficult to palpate; it may fade in and out and is easily obliterated with pressure.

+2: Pulse is difficult to palpate and may be obliterated with pressure so that light palpation is necessary. Once located, however, it is stronger than +1.

+3: Pulse is easily palpable, does not fade in and out, and is not easily obliterated by pressure. This pulse is considered to have normal volume.

+4: Pulse is strong, bounding, or hyperactive, easily palpated, and not obliterated with pressure. In some cases, such as aortic regurgitation, it is considered pathologic (1).

As the premedication effects subside, the child will become hungry. Begin the diet with clear liquids until no further effects of the premedication are evident. Then advance to a regular diet. The older the patient, the more likely vomiting would occur as a side effect of the premedication.

An ideal clear liquid is a light-colored, sugared carbonated drink that has been opened and set aside to allow the bubbles to disappear. Pour this over ice and let the child sip it. A sweet beverage such as this is generally better tolerated than water.

The morning after catheterization, the dressing is removed. A slight soreness is felt in the wound area. There are no restrictions on the child's activities. The parents should be taught the signs of infection (redness, swelling, tenderness, or pus from wound site) and the importance of contacting their pediatrician or cardiologist if infection occurs.

Interpretation: The common congenital cardiac defects will be listed in alphabetical order with anatomy, hemodynamics, and catheterization data explained for each defect. This information may be compared to the normal values in the heart diagram (Fig. 4-3).

Aortic Stenosis: Aortic stenosis (AS) is an obstruction at the aortic valve level interfering with the left ventricular (LV) outflow of blood. The obstruction may be in the valve itself, subaortic (below the valve), or supraaortic (above the valve). If it occurs at the valvular level, the valve may be bicuspid (two leaflets).

Catheterization data indicating aortic stenosis would show a difference in the systolic reading of the left ventricular and aortic (Ao) pressures. The difference would indicate the severity of stenosis. The dye injection in the left ventricle would outline the hypertrophied area causing the stenosis.

Atrial Septal Defect: Atrial septal defect (ASD) is an abnormal opening between the two atria. The defect allows left-to-right shunting of oxygenated blood at the atrial level. Catheterization data indicating an atrial septal defect show a rise in the oxygen saturation in the right atrium (RA) as compared to the superior vena caval (SVC) saturation. Also, in most cases, the catheter would easily pass through the hole from the right atrium to the left atrium (LA). The dye injection in the left atrium would show the left-to-right shunting of blood between the atria.

Coarctation of the Aorta: Coarctation of the aorta is a narrowing of the aorta. This narrowing can be located anywhere along the aorta, but is most commonly at the area where the ductus arteriosus attaches.

Catheterization data indicating a coarctation would be indicated by a systolic pressure difference along and across the narrowed area. The dye injection in the aorta would outline the narrowed area.

Endocardial Cushion Defect: The endocardial cushion is the area in the middle of the heart that forms the lower border of the atrial septum, the upper border of the ventricular septum, and the middle portions of the tricuspid and mitral valves. An endocardial cushion defect is an abnormal opening that may be complete, affecting all four areas. Usually the defect is incomplete, affecting the atrial and ventricular septums and the mitral valve.

Catheterization data indicate increased oxygen saturations in the right atrium and right ventricle. The pulmonary pressure is usually increased due to the left-to-right shunting at both levels. The dye injection into the left ventricle shows a left-to-right shunt from the left ventricle, mostly to the right atrium.

Patent Ductus Arteriosus: A patent ductus arteriosus (PDA) results from the failure of a fetal connection to close after birth. In fetal circulation, the ductus arteriosus connects the pulmonary artery to the aorta.

Catheterization data indicating a PDA would show an increase in pulmonary artery (PA) oxygen saturation due to the left-to-right shunting of oxygenated blood from the aorta. Often the catheter can be passed up the pulmonary artery, through the PDA, and down the aorta. Dye injection into the aorta shows blood shunting down the PDA to the pulmonary artery.

Pulmonary Stenosis: Pulmonary stenosis (PS) is an obstruction at the pulmonary valve level interfering with the right ventricular outflow of blood. The obstruction can be at the valve itself or subpulmonic (below the valve). Subpulmonic stenosis is generally referred to as infundibular stenosis. Infundibulum is the muscle area below the pulmonary artery valve. The pulmonary artery may be narrowed close to the valve or out into the lungs.

Catheterization data indicating pulmonary stenosis is shown in the difference in systolic pressure between the right ventricle and the pulmonary artery. The difference would indicate the severity of stenosis. The dye injection into the right ventricle would show the hypertrophied or narrowed areas.

Tetralogy of Fallot: Tetralogy of Fallot (TOF) is a term coined by Dr. Fallot who noted a number of cyanotic children with similar heart defects. These defects appeared in four groups: pulmonary stenosis, right ventricular hypertrophy of the infundibular region, ventricular septal defect, and overriding of the aorta. This means that the right ventricle has two outflow obstructions and that the unoxygenated blood can pass more easily through the ventricular septal defect and out the overriding aorta, causing the child to become cyanotic.

Catheterization data indicating TOF is shown by a pressure difference between the systolic reading of the right ventricle and pulmonary artery. Frequently the catheter more easily enters the wide open aorta instead of the stenosed pulmonary artery. The oxygen saturations in the aorta would be decreased due to the blood shunting right to left through the VSD. The dye injections would show this shunting, the stenosis, the hypertrophy, and the overriding of the aorta.

Transposition of the Great Arteries: Transposition of the great arteries (TGA) refers to the reversal of pulmonary artery and the aorta. The aorta empties the right ventricle. Thus, unoxygenated blood from the body comes into the right ventricle and empties back to the body out the aorta. The pulmonary artery empties the left ventricle. Red oxygenated blood comes from the lungs into the left ventricle and empties back to the lungs out the pulmonary artery. Thus, there are two complete separate circulations.

Emergency catheterization data are obtained. TGA is indicated by a marked decrease in oxygen saturations in the right atrium and right ventricle. The dye injection into the right ventricle shows the emptying into the aorta.

After the diagnosis of TGA is confirmed by catheterization, a special balloon catheter is passed through the foramen ovale in the atrial septum. The balloon is inflated in the left atrium and rapidly withdrawn through the foramen to the right atrium, rupturing the membrane covering the foramen. This provides a hole for oxygenated blood from the left atrium to pass to the right atrium, then down to the right ventricle, and out the aorta to the body. This is known as a balloon atrial septostomy and is only a palliative procedure.

Ventricular Septal Defect: Ventricular septal defect (VSD) is an abnormal opening between the two ventricles.

The defect allows left-to-right shunting of oxygenated blood at the ventricular level. Catheterization data indicating a VSD would be shown by a rise in the oxygen saturation in the right ventricle as compared to the oxygen saturation right atrium. A dye injection into the left ventricle would show the left-to-right shunting at the ventricular level.

REFERENCE

1. Miller KM, "Assessing Peripheral Perfusion." *Am J Nurs* 78:1673, 1978.

BIBLIOGRAPHY

Matthew UF (ed): *Manual of Pediatric Nursing Careplans.* Boston, Little, Brown & Co, 1979 pp 75–76.

Miller KM, "Assessing Peripheral Perfusion," *Am J Nurs* 78:1673–74, 1978.

Moss AJ, Adams FH, Emmanouilides GD: *Heart Disease in Infants, Children, and Adolescents,* ed 2. Baltimore, The Williams & Wilkins Co, 1977, pp 107–128.

Personal experience of the staff cardiologist at Childrens' Medical Center, Dallas, Texas, and this chapter's author.

Petrillo M, Sanger S: *Emotional Care of Hospitalized Children, an Environmental Approach.* Philadelphia & Toronto, JB Lippincott Co, 1972, pp 173–77.

Zander KS, Bower KA, Foster SD (eds): *Practical Manual for Patient-Teaching.* St Louis The C V Mosby Co, 1978, pp 29–46, 73.

Sacksteder S, Gildea JH, Dassey C: "Common Congenital Cardiac Defects," *Am J Nurs* 78:266–82, 1978.

Silver HK, Kempe CH, Bruyn HB: *Handbook of Pediatrics,* ed 10. Los Altos, Ca, Lange Medical Publications, 1973, p 214.

Taber CW: *Taber's Cyclopedic Medical Dictionary,* ed 10. Philadelphia, F A David Company, 1965, p C-21.

5

Pulmonary Diagnostic Procedures

BLOOD GAS ANALYSIS

Blood gas analysis is an invasive procedure that provides measurements of oxygen, carbon dioxide, and hydrogen in the arterial blood. Blood gas measurements effectively provide an estimate of pulmonary oxygen transport, alveolar ventilation, and the net acid-base status of the blood (1).

Arterial puncture is the method most commonly used for blood gas analysis, although venous blood samples may be used to measure pH and carbon dioxide content.

Premedication: None.

Diet: No restriction.

Time: 2 to 3 minutes.

Procedure: A 1 cc gas-tight syringe, fitted with a 25 gauge needle, is prepared by drawing up sufficient heparin to wet the plunger and fill the dead space of the syringe and the needle. The excess heparin is expelled with the syringe in an upright position. An artery (brachial or radial) is selected, the overlying skin is cleansed with 1% iodine, and the iodine solution is removed with alcohol. With the palpating finger immobilizing the artery, the needle is directed into the artery with the bevel up. Aspiration with the plunger is not necessary; the syringe will fill with blood when the artery is entered. A large volume is unnecessary since the blood PO_2, PCO_2, and pH can be measured from as little as 0.1 ml. After the blood sample has been obtained, the needle is quickly withdrawn and firm pressure held on the puncture site for at least 5 minutes. The syringe is tightly capped, submerged in a beaker of ice, and taken to the laboratory for immediate analysis. Delay in performing determinations after collection of the sample causes inaccurate results; if the blood is kept at room temperature, the pH drops and the PCO_2 rises as a result of metabolism of the cellular elements in the syringe. Such changes are minimal if the blood is stored on ice, allowing accurate determinations up to 2 hours later with only a slight fall in pH (less than 0.015 unit) (2). Exposure of the sample to room air must be avoided, because the PCO_2 and PO_2 will tend to equilibrate with the atmosphere, resulting in inaccurate values. Inspired oxygen concentration ($F_I O_2$) and any elevation of body temperature should be reported to the laboratory when the blood sample is sent.

Preparation: No physical preparation is necessary. The child should understand the importance of holding still during the procedure. He will feel a stick and then pain for a moment until the required amount of blood fills the syringe. The needle then will be quickly withdrawn and firm pressure applied to the area for 10 to 15 minutes.

Aftercare: Firm pressure must be held on the puncture site for at least 10 to 15 minutes to prevent hematoma formation. The extremity should be observed for arteriospasm indicated by pallor or coolness distal to the puncture site. After all bleeding has stopped, arteriospasm may be relieved by the application of warm compresses. Any complication should be reported to the physician immediately.

Interpretation of Findings: See Appendix B for normal values.

BRONCHOGRAPHY

Bronchography is an invasive procedure in which a radio-paque material is instilled into the trachea and bronchi through a catheter of nebulizer, permitting x-ray film visualization of the entire tracheobronchial tree. Broncho-grams are useful for evaluating congenital defects or airway problems that have resulted in damaged pulmonary structures (bronchiectasis).

Premedication: The child receives an IM medication 45 minutes to an hour before the procedure. The medications usually ordered are atropine to minimize secretions and a narcotic analgesic to sedate the child and potentiate the anesthetic.

Diet: The child is kept NPO at least 4 hours before the bronchoscopy to prevent vomiting and possible aspiration of gastric contents.

Consent: An authorization signed by the parent or guard-ian is necessary.

Time: 1 hour.

Procedure: Bronchography may be performed under general or local anesthesia.
   General anesthesia, although more comfortable for the child, has the disadvantages of suppressing the cough reflex and depressing respiration. Before intubation is performed, an IV is started and a satisfactory plane of anesthesia achieved by inhalation of an anesthetic gas or infusion of an anesthetic drug.
   Local laryngeal anesthesia is accomplished by swabbing and/or spraying the throat and larynx with a topical anesthetic. Since cough and gag reflexes are stimulated, the child needs support and restraint at this time.

Once general or local anesthesia is accomplished, an endotracheal airway is inserted and an opaque catheter passed down the tube under fluoroscopic control. A small amount of contrast medium is then injected and, if awake, the patient is instructed to inhale deeply to spread the contrast material throughout the lung. The child is tilted into various positions, which causes the liquid contrast material to run along the walls of the entire tracheobronchial tree. A series of spot films are taken, guided by what is seen fluoroscopically. The child is instructed to cough in order to expectorate the contrast material, and posttussive x-rays films are taken. Usually the lungs are examined separately, particularly if pulmonary function is abnormal.

An alternative method of introducing the contrast material is through nebulization. The conscious child can inhale nebulized Dionosil or tantalum powder*. Ultrasonic nebulizers deliver particles of contrast material of the appropriate size to reach the small airways (3).

Preparation: The child should receive thorough oral hygiene the evening before and the morning of the procedure. The mouth may be inspected at this time for any loose teeth that may become dislodged during the procedure. Postural drainage may be ordered the morning before the procedure to clear the bronchi of secretions that would interfere with filling by the radiopaque material.

The child should be prepared for the IM premedication and the drowsy feeling following it. If bronchography is to be performed under general anesthetic, the child should be told he will be asleep during the procedure and will awake in the "wake-up room." He should also be told when he will be returned to his own room, where his parents will be, and when he will be able to resume his normal diet and activities.

---

*At the time of this writing tantalum has not yet been approved by the FDA for widespread use in humans.

If the procedure is to be performed under local anesthesia, the child should be prepared for the uncomfortable swabbing and/or spraying of his throat and larynx that will stimulate cough and gag reflexes. The bitter-tasting anesthetic will make his tongue and throat feel swollen. He will feel as if he is unable to swallow, so he should let the saliva run out of his mouth into a tissue or an emesis basin that will be provided.

Since relaxation allows the procedure to be performed more rapidly and more comfortably, the child should be made to understand its importance. He should be reassured that he will be able to breathe while the instruments are in his throat since the endotracheal tube is hollow. Breathing exercises are helpful and can be mastered even by small children. For example, the child can practice breathing through his mouth only, with his mouth open, and then through his nose only with his mouth open (4). Practice in coughing and deep breathing is essential. If the contrast material is to be instilled with a nebulizer, the child should be allowed to practice breathing through the equipment before the procedure. Postural drainage may be done after bronchography, and a preprocedural practice session can be most helpful.

The child should be told that he will not be given anything to eat or drink for several hours after the procedure until his throat "wakes up." He may have a slight sore throat for several hours.

Restraint Necessary: If general anesthesia is not used, the small child may be effectively restrained by secure wrapping. Sedation and reassurance are usually adequate to control most older children during the procedure except for the application of the local anesthetic. During this uncomfortable portion of the procedure the child will need firm restraint.

Aftercare: The child should be allowed to recover from general anesthesia or sedation in a protected environment.

To prevent aspiration the child should be placed on his side and kept NPO until a normal gag reflex has returned.

The child should be encouraged to cough to clear the bronchial tree of contrast material. Postural drainage may also be indicated.

The child should be watched closely for symptoms of laryngospasm or laryngeal edema. The child's temperature should be checked regularly, since the contrast material may block small airways, causing atelectasis.

BRONCHOSCOPY

Bronchoscopy is an invasive procedure through which the interior of the tracheobronchial tree can be directly visualized. In addition to its obvious diagnostic value, bronchoscopy is an ideal means for removing foreign bodies from the major airways or obtaining a biopsy specimen. Bronchoscopy can be performed with either a rigid or a flexible fiberoptic scope. The standard rigid bronchoscope (Fig. 5-1) permits visualization down to the orifices of the lower lobe segmental bronchi. Newer pediatric rigid bronchoscopes are now equipped with fiberoptic illumination and improved telescopic lens systems that allow effective examination of even small infants*. Exploration of the smaller airways and upper lobe bronchi is made possible by the flexible bronchofiberscope (Fig. 5-2). Although the flexible bronchofiberscope revolutionized adult pulmonary medicine, its use in pediatrics has serious limitations, primarily because of the space occupation of the airway. The patient must breathe around (rather than through) the flexible bronchoscope. Another drawback inherent in flexible pediatric bronchoscopes (3 ml) is that they are too

---

*The bronchofiberscope operates in a manner similar to other fiberoptic scopes. See "Upper GI Endoscopy" for further explanation.

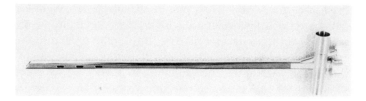

Figure 5-1
Rigid bronchoscope.

small to accommodate channels for irrigation, suction, or passage of brushes or biopsy forceps. For these reasons, use of the flexible bronchoscope is impractical in infants and children under the age of approximately 8 years (5). The larger fiberscope may be used in children 10 years old or older. The flexible bronchofiberscope may also be used in conjunction with a rigid scope.

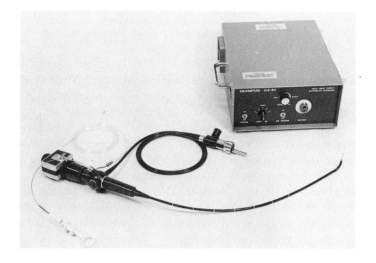

Figure 5-2
Flexible bronchofiberscope. (Photograph courtesy of Olympus Corporation of America, New Hyde Park, New York.)

Premedication: Bronchoscopy is usually performed under general anesthesia, in which case the child would receive a routine preoperative medication 30 to 45 minutes before the procedure. However, fiberoptic bronchoscopy with local anesthesia and sedation is advocated by some (6,7). An IM injection of a narcotic analgesic or sedative is usually given an hour before a bronchoscopy is performed under local anesthesia. In addition to increasing relaxation and alleviating coughing and gagging, premedication with atropine decreases bronchial secretions, relaxes the bronchial smooth muscle, and decreases the risk of postbronchoscopy laryngospasm.

Diet: The child is kept NPO at least 4 hours before the procedure to prevent vomiting and possible aspiration of gastric contents.

Consent: An authorization signed by the parent or guardian is necessary.

Time: 15 minutes. Usually another 15 minutes is required for the induction of general anesthesia.

Procedure: If general anesthesia is used, an IV infusion is started and the child is connected to an electrocardiographic monitor. General anesthesia is induced. If local anesthesia is used, the mouth, pharynx, and hypopharynx are sprayed with Cetacaine or a similar agent. Additional anesthetic may be administered by a gargle or transtracheally by needle. Usually, adequate local anesthesia is obtained in 10 to 15 minutes. If a rigid bronchoscope is used, the child is placed in a dorsal recumbent position with his neck extended and his head slightly elevated. The head may be moved from side to side after the bronchoscope enters the trachea to ease the passage into the two main bronchi. With a flexible bronchoscope, the child may be sitting or lying down; special positioning is not necessary. The bronchoscope is passed through the child's mouth, larynx, and vocal cords, and into the trachea. The trachea and bronchi are inspected and the carina is checked for position and mobility. Foreign bodies or mucus plugs may be removed. The patient's color, pulse, and respiration are carefully monitored throughout the procedure, since dangerous hypoxemia may occur (7).

Preparation: Platelet count, prothrombin time, partial thromboplastin time, and bleeding time should be obtained before the bronchoscopy, particularly if biopsy is planned (see Appendix B for normal values). The mouth should be inspected for loose teeth.

The child should be given a simple explanation of the procedure. If general anesthesia is to be used, the child should be prepared for the IM preoperative medication and the drowsy feeling following it. He should be told that he will be asleep during the procedure and will experience no discomfort during that time. He will awaken in the "wake-up room" with an IV infusion and will be returned to his own room when he is fully awake. The IV will be removed after he is fully awake and taking fluids. He should also be prepared for suctioning and postural drainage following bronchoscopy and should be told that he may experience a sore throat and cough for a day or so. It is also important to teach the child how to breathe using the abdominal and diaphragmatic muscles and how to cough properly.

If local anesthesia with sedation is planned, the child must be adequately prepared for this potentially frightening procedure. Application of the local anesthetic is the most uncomfortable part of the procedure since the cough and gag reflexes are stimulated. Cetacaine or a similar agent is sprayed in the mouth, pharynx, and hypopharynx. Additional anesthetic may be administered by gargle or transtracheally by needle. Usually, adequate anesthesia is obtained in 10 to 15 minutes. The child will feel as though his tongue and throat are swollen and that he is unable to swallow. Secretions will be suctioned throughout the procedure. The bronchoscope is introduced when local anesthesia has been achieved. The child should be reassured that he will be able to breathe while the tube is in his throat and that he will not suffocate or choke. He should be told that he should try to breathe normally during the examination, instead of holding his breath. He must understand the importance of relaxing and remaining still. The child will feel pressure as the scope passes through his mouth and larynx, but he will not feel pain. The child should be warned that the procedure will be done in a darkened room so that the doctor can see more clearly the structures lighted by the scope. The doctor and his assistants will be wearing masks and gloves. The child should also be told that his eyes will be covered during the procedure to protect them. The scope will be removed when the examination is completed. The child may have fluids when normal swallowing reflexes have returned, usually about 2 hours after the procedure. The child will feel very sleepy for several hours until the sedative wears off. The child should also be prepared to expect the mist tent in which he will be placed after bronchoscopy. A practice session in the "plastic house" or tent before the procedure is helpful. The child should also be prepared for postural drainage after the procedure if it is anticipated.

Restraint Necessary: If general anesthesia is not used, the younger child is most effectively restrained by wrapping him in sheets in such a way that complete freedom of motion of the chest is permitted. In this way the child does not have a feeling of suffocation but is safely immobilized.

The older child is usually able to remain still with gentle restraint if given adequate support and explanation.

Aftercare: The child should be allowed to recover from anesthesia in a protected environment. Oral intake is withheld until normal swallowing and bowel sounds have returned. Once the gag reflex has returned, generous fluids help to decrease throat soreness and aid in mobilizing secretions. Usually the child is placed in a mist tent after bronchoscopy to lessen laryngeal edema. Careful suctioning and postural drainage may also be necessary. Efforts should be made to promote comfort and minimize crying.

The child should be closely observed for complications such as hemorrhage and respiratory distress (laryngospasm or laryngeal edema), which are indicated by changes in vital signs and observations and by changes in behavior. The physician should be notified immediately in case of laryngeal stridor, dyspnea, retractions, or shortness of breath. The child's sputum should be observed for indications of hemorrhage. Slightly blood-streaked sputum is normal after biopsy, but frank bleeding must be reported immediately.

DIRECT LARYNGOSCOPY

Direct laryngoscopy is an invasive procedure that provides visualization of the larynx. The laryngoscope is a hollow, rigid metal tube, lighted at its distal end by batteries (Fig. 5-3).

Laryngoscopy is valuable for inspection of the larynx, especially for evaluation of laryngeal stridor, removal of foreign bodies, determination of the presence of inflammation, or insertion of an endotracheal tube.

Premedication: If performed under general anesthesia, an IM preoperative medication may be given 45 minutes before the procedure.

Diet: The child should be kept NPO for 3 hours before the procedure if possible.

Time: 15 minutes.

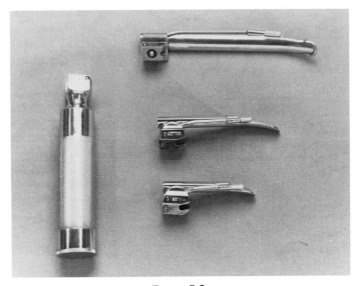

Figure 5-3
Laryngoscope with 3 Miller blades.

Procedure: Either local or general anesthesia may be used. (Refer to "Bronchoscopy" for anesthesia.) The patient is placed in a dorsal recumbent position, the head slightly extended with the jaw thrust forward. A folded towel or a small flat pillow may be placed under the head, but excessive extension is to be avoided. The head should be held in the "sniffing" position with a midline alignment of the mouth, pharynx, larynx, and trachea. The laryngoscope is passed into the right side of the mouth and down to the larynx under direct vision. The illuminated larynx is then examined. Biopsy or removal of foreign objects may be performed through the laryngoscope. An endotracheal tube may be passed between the vocal cords under direct vision.

Preparation: Refer to "Bronchoscopy." The batteries and

light in the laryngoscope should be checked before the
procedure.

Restraint Necessary: Refer to "Bronchoscopy."

Aftercare: Refer to "Bronchoscopy."

LUNG PUNCTURE

Lung puncture is an invasive procedure that is used to
obtain a sample of lung exudate for examination. This
technique provides data about the causative agents in
pneumonia, yielding accurate information not otherwise
easily obtained. Lung puncture is used in the critically ill
child for whom identification of the causative organism is
particularly important to guide treatment, if a causative
organism cannot be isolated by a simpler means, and when
pneumonia complicates the treatment course in a child
with altered host defense mechanisms (8).

Premedication: None.

Diet: No restriction.

Consent: An authorization signed by the parent or guardian is necessary.

Time: 10 minutes.

Procedure: The child is held in a sitting position, or if
the upper lobes are involved the child is restrained prone
or supine. The puncture site is determined by the area of
greatest consolidation as shown on an x-ray film. The site
is cleansed with an antiseptic solution, and it is anesthetized
with 2% procaine hydrochloride down to the pleura. The
areas of the heart, great vessels, and liver are avoided. A

20 or 21 gauge needle is attached to a 10 ml syringe that contains 1 ml of sterile isotonic saline solution*. The needle is quickly inserted to a depth of 3 or 4 cm and gentle suction is applied by withdrawing the plunger of the syringe. A Band-Aid is put over the puncture site. The aspirated contents are cultured immediately and appropriately stained. During the procedure the child's color, pulse, and respiration should be watched carefully.

Preparation: No physical preparation is necessary.

The child should be given a simple explanation of the procedure and be prepared for a cold feeling when the skin is cleansed with an antiseptic solution, a stinging sensation when the area is infiltrated with local anesthetic, and pressure when the needle is inserted into the pleura. The needle will remain in the chest only a few seconds, and little pain should be felt after injection of the local anesthetic. (Occasionally, pain may be felt when the needle passes the parietal pleura even after local anesthetic has been injected.)

The child should be helped to understand the importance of remaining still during the procedure.

Restraint Necessary: It is imperative that the child remain still during the injection of the local anesthetic and during aspiration. Sudden movement could force the needle through the pleural space, damaging the pleura and/or lung. Gentle, firm restraint and a calm, reassuring manner are most important. Infants may be held against the assistant's chest in the "burping" position. Older children should sit on the treatment table supported by an assistant. If the erect position is not possible, the recumbent position most adaptable to removal of fluid may be used.

Aftercare: Vital signs should be checked frequently for

---

*It is essential that the saline contain no bacteriostatic agent, or culture results will be inaccurate.

several hours after lung puncture. Complications of lung puncture are rare, but pneumothorax and transient hemoptysis have been reported (8,9). A chest x-ray film may be obtained after the procedure to check for pneumothorax. The puncture site should be checked for bleeding. Coughing, hemoptysis, or significant changes in color or vital signs should be reported.

PULMONARY FUNCTION TESTS

Pulmonary function tests are noninvasive procedures used for the evaluation of lung volumes and flow rates. Such tests are useful in differentiating restrictive (e.g., respiratory muscle weakness) and obstructive (e.g., asthma, cystic fibrosis) lung disease. Pulmonary function tests do not provide a specific diagnosis but are valuable in assessing the severity of specific diseases and in evaluating treatment.

Premedication: None.

Diet: No restrictions.

Time: Time required to perform pulmonary function tests varies with the number of measurements and the child's ability to cooperate.

Procedure: The child is made comfortable, either sitting or standing, next to the spirometer*. Nose clips are applied, and the child is instructed to breathe normally through the mouthpiece, closing his lips tightly to prevent air leaks. After the child has mastered breathing through

---

*The spirometer is used to measure tidal volume, respiratory rate, vital capacity, inspiratory capacity, and expiratory reserve volume.

the mouthpiece, he is asked to breathe in as deeply as possible, hold it for at least 3 seconds, and then blow into the mouthpiece as hard, fast, and long as he can (Blow! Push! *Push! PUSH!*). Usually, several efforts are made and the best one is recorded. Both lung volumes and flow rates may be measured.

Lung Volumes and Compartments: There are four primary volumes:

- Tidal volume (TV): the volume of air inhaled or exhaled with each breath during quiet breathing.
- Residual volume (RV): the volume of air remaining in the lungs after maximal exhalation.
- Expiratory reserve volume (ERV): the maximal volume of air exhaled from the end-expiratory level.
- Inspiratory reserve volume (IRV): the maximal volume of air inhaled from the end-inspiratory level.

There are also four capacities. Each of these capacities includes more than one of the volumes.

- Vital capacity (VC): the maximal volume of air exhaled from the point of maximum inspiration (VC = TV + IRV + ERV).
- Inspiratory capacity (IC): the maximal volume of air that can be expired from the end-expiratory level (IC = TV + IRV).
- Functional residual capacity (FRC): the volume of air remaining in the lungs at the end-expiratory position (FRC = ERV + RV).
- Total lung capacity (TLC): the sum of all volume compartments or the volume of air in the lungs after maximal inspiration (TLC = TV + IRV + ERV + RV).

Functional residual capacity, residual volume, and total lung capacity are measured by one of the following indirect methods:

1. Open-circuit nitrogen washout method: The child breathes 100% oxygen, usually for 7 minutes, to "wash out" all of the nitrogen from the lungs. The expired air is collected and measured for nitrogen concentration. Since alveolar air is known to contain 80% nitrogen, the total amount of air in the lungs can be computed. A significantly prolonged nitrogen washout time indicates an obstructive disease.

2. Closed-circuit helium dilution method: The child rebreathes a mixture of helium (an inert, relatively insoluble gas) and air from a spirometer until the concentration of the two gases is equal in both the lungs and the spirometer. The new concentration of helium is recorded. Since the initial volume of helium is unchanged, the initial volume of gas in the lungs can be calculated.

3. Total body plethysmograph method: The child is placed in the plethysmograph or "body box" (Fig. 5-4) and the door is shut, forming an airtight system. Based on Boyle's law, the volumes of gas in the lung can be computed as the child breathes, varying pressure within the chamber.

The nitrogen and helium methods measure only gas in communication with the airways. The plethysmograph method is a more accurate and rapid measurement in obstructive disease. It also permits measurement of airway resistance. All three methods can be used effectively with children 7 or 8 years of age or older (10).

Flow Rates (ventilation tests):

- Forced vital capacity (FVC): the largest volume of gas that can be forcefully and rapidly exhaled from the lungs, starting from maximal inspiration and ending with maximal expiration.
- Timed, forced expiratory volume (FEV): the amount of

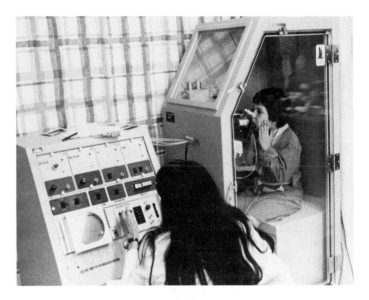

Figure 5-4
Plethysmography chamber.

air that can be forced out of fully inflated lungs in a given time. Usually, the FEV per second is measured. FEV 1/FVC is the ratio of forced expiratory volume in 1 second divided by the forced vital capacity. This is expressed as a percentage.

- Peak expiratory flow rate (PEFR): the most rapid flow of gas during a forced expiration, expressed in terms of 1 minute (liters per minute). PEFR may be viewed as a quantitative measure of cough effectiveness (10).

Preparation: The pulmonary function laboratory should be notified of the time when the child last received a bronchodilator, mucolytic agent, postural drainage, or any other treatment affecting respiratory function. Optimal pulmonary function results depend on the understanding and cooperation of the child. Preparation should include practice periods in which the child becomes familiar with the equipment. He should practice breathing through the mouthpiece and with the nose clip in place and become accustomed to the plethysmography chamber. The child must also learn to perform a maximal vital capacity maneuver, which consists of full inspiration, a brief breath hold, and a sudden sustained maximal expiratory effort. The young child may be taught this procedure by playing "make believe it's your birthday. You have to blow out all the candles with only one breath." If the practice is made into a game, it can be fun and the child will be more willing to cooperate. Usually, children younger than 10 years old perform better if they are standing, but older children seem to perform equally well either sitting or standing during the procedure.

Because pulmonary function testing requires that the child understand, cooperate, and exert himself, adequate preparation is essential. Forced vital capacity (FVC) and forced expiratory volume (FEV) can be measured accurately in children as young as 5 years old. Even younger children can perform satisfactory (PEFR) tests (10).

Recent developments in apparatus and technique have made possible measurements of pulmonary function in infants and children under 5 years of age. Only functional residual capacity (FRC) can be measured accurately in this age group. Body plethysmography is the simplest method for obtaining FRC. A tight-fitting face mask may be used, but since the respiratory drive is very sensitive to facial stimulation, this method may produce erroneous results (11). Indirect measurements such as electrical impedance and determination of chest movement can be used to obtain minute volume and crying vital capacity (12).

Aftercare: No physical aftercare is necessary.

Interpretation of Findings: Although a comprehensive discussion of interpretation of pulmonary function tests is beyond the scope of this text, a few pertinent facts will be presented:

- Vital capacity becomes decreased in both restrictive and obstructive disease.
- Total lung capacity becomes decreased in restrictive disease and tends to increase in obstructive disease.
- A significantly low forced vital capacity is usually interpreted as a restrictive impairment.
- A significantly low forced expiratory volume may be produced either by restrictive or obstructive disease.
- A significantly low FEV/VC is interpreted as obstructive.
- A significantly low peak expiratory flow rate is usually interpreted as obstructive disease, especially if vital capacity is normal, but lesser reductions in PEFR may also occur in restrictive disease.*

REFERENCES

1. Petty TL: *Pulmonary Diagnostic Techniques.* Philadelphia, Lea & Febiger, 1975.
2. Korones SB: *High-Risk Newborn Infants.* St Louis, CV Mosby Co, 1977.
3. Johnston RF: *Pulmonary Care.* New York, Grune & Stratton, Inc, 1972.
4. Luckmann, J, Sorensen KC: *Medical-Surgical Nursing.* Philadelphia, WB Saunders Co, 1974.
5. Hyde RW: New Pulmonary Diagnostic Procedures. *Am J Dis Child* 126:292, 1973.
6. Atkins JP: Bronchoscopic Problems of Infancy and Childhood. *Arch Otolaryngol* 79:152, 1964.
7. Kendig EL (ed): *Disorders of the Respiratory Tract in Children* 126:292, 1973.
8. Hughes JR, Sinha DP, Cooper MR, et al: Lung Tap in Childhood. *Pediatrics* 44:486–492, 1969.

*Interpretation of findings was adapted from the National Cystic Fibrosis Research Foundation publication *Source Book in Pediatric Pulmonary Disease.*

9. Mimica I, Donoso E, Howard J, et al: Lung Puncture in the Etiological Diagnosis of Pneumonia. *Am J Dis Child* 122:278, 1971.
10. National Cystic Fibrosis Research Foundation. *Source Book in Pediatric Pulmonary Disease.* Atlanta, Ga, September 1971.
11. Hatch DJ, Milner AD: The Measurement of Lung Function in Infants and Children Under Five Years of Age. *Int Anesthesiol Clin* 12:37, 1974.
12. Kempe CH, Silver HK, O'Brien D: *Current Pediatric Diagnosis and Treatment.* Los Altos, Ca, Lange Medical Publications, 1974.

BIBLIOGRAPHY

Atkins, JP: Bronchoscopic Problems of Infancy and Childhood. *Arch Otolaryngol* 79:152, 1964.

Chernick V, Avery ME: *Disorders of the Respiratory Tract in Children,* ed 3, Kendig EL, Jr (ed). Philadelphia, WB Saunders Co, 1977.

Ferguson CF, Kendig EL: *Pediatric Otolaryngology,* Vol II. Philadelphia, WB Saunders Co, 1972.

Gans SL, Berci G: Advances in Endoscopy of Infants and Children. *J Pediatr Surg* 6:199, 1971.

Hatch DJ, Milner AD: The Management of Lung Function in Infants and Children Under Five Years of Age. *Int Clinics* 12:37, 1974.

Hughes JR, Sinha BP, Cooper MR, et al: Lung Tap in Childhood. *Pediatrics* 44:486–492, 1969.

Hyde RW: New Pulmonary Diagnostic Procedure. *Am J Dis Child* 126:292, 1973.

Johnston RF: *Pulmonary Care.* New York, Grune & Stratton, Inc, 1972.

Jona JZ, Belin RP: Fiberoptic Bronchoscopy in Infants and Children: Advances and Clinical Usage. *J Ky Med Assoc,* September 1975, p 485.

Kempe CH, Silver HK, O'Brien D: *Current Pediatric Diagnosis and Treatment.* Los Altos, Ca, Lange Medical Publications, 1974.

Kendig EL (ed): *Disorders of the Respiratory Tract in Children.* Philadelphia, WB Saunders Co, 1977.

Klein JO: Diagnostic Lung Puncture in the Pneumonias of Infants and Children. *Pediatrics* 44:486, 1969.

Kock MA: *Dynamic Bronchoscopy.* New York, Springer-Verlag New York, Inc, 1977.

Korones SB: *High Risk Newborn Infants.* St Louis, CV Mosby Co, 1977.

Luckmann J, Sorensen KC: *Medical-Surgical Nursing.* Philadelphia, WB Saunders Co, 1974.

Mimica I, Donoso E, Howard J, et al: Lung Puncture in the Etiological Diagnosis of Pneumonia. *Am J Dis Child* 122:278, 1971.

National Cystic Fibrosis Research Foundation. *Source Book in Pediatric Pulmonary Disease.* Atlanta, Ga, September 1971.

Petty TL: *Pulmonary Diagnostic Techniques.* Philadelphia, Lea & Febiger, 1975.

Poradowska W, Reszke S, Kubicz S: *Surgical Lung Diseases in Childhood.* Warsaw, Polish Medical Publisher, 1972.

Stradling P: *Diagnostic Bronchoscopy,* ed 3. New York, Churchill Livingston, 1976.

Wood RE, Fink RJ: Applications of Flexible Fiberoptic Bronchoscopes in Infants and Children. *Chest* 73(suppl 737):5, 1978.

6

Neurologic Diagnostic Procedures

CEREBRAL ANGIOGRAPHY

Cerebral angiography is an invasive procedure in which a radiopaque substance is injected into an artery, providing x-ray film visualization of the brain's vascular system. Angiography is useful in identifying vascular anomalies or lesions large enough to grossly distort the cerebral vascular system. This procedure is often preferred to air studies (i.e, pneumoencephalography, ventriculography) because it has a lower mortality rate and is less traumatizing (1).

Contraindications to cerebral angiography include allergy to the contrast medium (especially iodine-based dyes), renal insufficiency, blood dyscrasias, or anticoagulant therapy (2).

Premedication: Because general anesthesia is usually given, a preoperative sedative is administered intramuscularly 20 to 30 minutes before the procedure.

Diet: The child is kept NPO 6 to 8 hours before the procedure.

Consent: An authorization signed by the parent or guardian is necessary.

Time: 30 minutes to 2 hours.

Procedure: General anesthesia is induced. A radiopaque substance is injected into a carotid, vertebral, femoral, or brachial artery or into a dural sinus. In smaller children surgical exposure of the vessel may be necessary. A series

115

of x-ray films are taken at rapid intervals from various angles. After the needle is removed, a sterile dressing is placed over the site and pressure maintained for 10 to 15 minutes to prevent bleeding and the formation of a hematoma. Throughout the procedure the child's cardiovascular status is observed closely.

Occasionally after injection, an intravenous pyelogram may also be recorded to discover unsuspected renal abnormalities.

Preparation: A clear, simple explanation of the procedure and its purpose should be given to the child and his parents. They should be prepared for the period of time the child will be NPO and for the preoperative medication. The child should also receive reassurance regarding general anesthesia. After the procedure the child may have an ice pack on the injection site and his vital signs and injection site will be checked frequently for a few hours.

The child's hair should be unbraided, unmatted, and free of anything that would produce extraneous shadows on the x-ray films. The child and/or parents should be questioned about any allergies to drugs, especially iodine, and seafood. Immediately before the procedure, baseline vital signs and neurological vital signs should be obtained and recorded. If a femoral puncture site is to be used, the pedal pulses of both feet should be checked and marked before the procedure. If a carotid or vertebral puncture is planned, the circumference of the neck should be measured and recorded. The level of the neck where the circumference was measured should be marked for later reference. (2).

Aftercare: The child should be kept comfortable and observed closely for complications. Vital signs are checked every 15 minutes for 1 hour and slowly tapered to every 4 hours for 24 hours. An ice pack is placed over the puncture site.

If a femoral puncture site was used, the leg should be

immobilized with a sandbag for at least 4 hours. The puncture site should be observed frequently for hematoma or bleeding. Pulses distal to the puncture site, color, and temperature of the extremity should be checked frequently to detect arterial occlusion. If the angiography was done by carotid or vertebral puncture, serial measurements of neck circumference may help to detect swelling. Rate and quality of respiration should also be noted. The physician should be notified if the child develops difficulty in breathing or swallowing, or if decreased hand grip or facial weakness appears on the side opposite the injection.

Arterial occlusions developing after angiography are surgical emergencies that, if untreated, may result in the loss of an extremity or severe stroke (2).

COMPUTERIZED TRANSAXIAL TOMOGRAPHY

Computerized transaxial tomography (CAT or EMI scan), lauded as the most effective neuroradiologic tool known, eliminates problems associated with many of the invasive contrast procedures such as pneumoencephalography and arteriography. CAT is noninvasive, is easy to perform, and does not require admission to the hospital. The most recent computerized tomographic units are capable of examining the whole body in addition to the head.

CAT works on the same principle as conventional radiology but with much greater precision and often less radiation exposure (3). The basic CAT brain scanner system consists of the scanning apparatus (the x-ray source and a sodium iodide crystal detector), a photomultiplier tube, a computer, and a cathode ray oscilloscope (4). The entire assembly, with the x-ray tube on one side of the child's head and the detectors on the other, moves synchronously past the patient in a straight line to obtain a series of radiation intensity measurements. At the completion of each 180-degree sweep, the entire assembly then moves vertically, repeating the motions until the entire head has been scanned. The information obtained from the readings is fed into a computer that reconstructs a two- or three-dimensional image from the one-dimensional projections. The processed information from the computer can be displayed in two ways: the data can be presented in digital form as a computerprinted digital map or as an oscilloscopic visualization in shades of gray that correspond to the density of tissue (5). High x-ray absorption values (e.g., bone) are printed as white, and low values (e.g., air) as black, just as in conventional x-ray films. Very small variations in absorption can be shown to reveal structures not visible on plain x-ray films such as ventricles, sulci, and blood clots (6). A Polaroid photograph is taken of the image for a permanent record. The total time for this procedure on the original CAT system was 20 minutes, but newer models have been introduced that accomplish this in 4 to 6 minutes. The CAT scan is a noninvasive procedure, but a water soluble iodized contrast medium may be injected intravenously to improve visualization of highly vascular lesions.

The CAT scan may be useful in the diagnosis of such conditions as abscesses, cysts, large aneurysms, subdural hematomas, vascular malformations, CVAs, and intracranial hemorrhages. CAT is often the preferred initial diagnostic procedure in suspected hydrocephalus and is accurate in the detection and precise localization of brain tumors (7).

Premedication: Small children may require sedation 20 to 30 minutes before the procedure in order to remain still since a very small amount of movement prevents accurate CAT scanning. Very ill or mentally handicapped children may need a general anesthetic.

Diet: No restriction necessary unless general anesthesia is planned. In that case the child should be kept NPO 4 to 6 hours before the procedure to prevent vomiting and possible aspiration of gastric contents.

Consent: An authorization signed by the parent or guardian is desirable, especially if a contrast medium is to be injected.

Time: 30 minutes.

Procedure: The child lies in a supine position on a couch, and the portion of the head to be studied is placed between the scanner and the photomultiplier. A strap (or rubber diaphragm in older units) is fitted snugly around the child's head, and restraints are applied since any motion will destroy the fine detail of a CAT scan. The scanner is rotated slowly 180 degrees around the child's head in several different planes. Readings are taken at each degree. Absorption coefficients* of tissues at different planes through the head are recorded.

When the scan is completed, the computer produces an image from the absorption coefficients presented. Photographs are taken of the image on the screen for a permanent record that can later be interpreted.

Preparation: If a contrast medium is to be used, the child should be checked for allergy to seafood or iodine. The procedure should be explained simply and clearly to the parents and child. They should understand that the CAT scan is painless and safe. The child must realize the necessity of remaining motionless during the procedure, which will last about 30 minutes. He should be told that

---

*Absorption coefficients are numbers assigned to different tissue densities ranging from −500 for air, 0 for water, +20 to +30 for normal brain, +80 for extravasated or clotted blood, and +500 for bone.

soft straps will be placed snugly around his head and body to help him hold still and to make a better picture. A description and picture of the equipment may help to allay the child's anxiety.

Restraint Necessary: The child must remain perfectly still during the CAT scan. Restraint may be provided by a padded head holder, adhesive head straps, and straps overlapping the trunk and extremities. Sedation may be helpful in small children.

Aftercare: No physical aftercare necessary.

ELECTROENCEPHALOGRAPHY

Electroencephalography (EEG) is a noninvasive procedure through which the electrical activity of the brain is recorded. An EEG may be performed to aid in the diagnosis and management of seizure disorders, to determine damaged or nonfunctioning areas*, to follow the progress of a child after a CNS infection or a head injury.

Premedication: If a sleep EEG is to be performed, a hypnotic or other drug may be indicated for use before the procedure. Usually, anticonvulsants are not discontinued before an EEG.

Diet: The child should not be given any coffee, tea, cola drinks, or alcohol on the day of the examination, since they contain stimulants or depressants and may alter brain

---

*Although EEGs are valuable in localizing tumors and the focal pattern of seizures in relation to the focus of the lesion, they are only a screening tool; they do not confirm the presence of lesions in the brain stem, ventricles, or suprasellar region (8).

wave activity. The child should not be kept without food for a long time before the test; hypoglycemia may modify the normal EEG pattern.

Time: 45 to 60 minutes for a routine EEG. Approximately 3 hours for a sleep EEG.

Procedure: With the child sitting in a chair or lying down, 16 electrodes are secured to his scalp with collodion or paste (Fig. 6-1). The electrodes are evenly distributed over the entire scalp. The electrode placement takes about 15 minutes.

The child is then instructed to lie quietly with his eyes closed (Fig. 6-2). An adult may help the child relax and fall asleep by sitting beside him, talking quietly, or telling

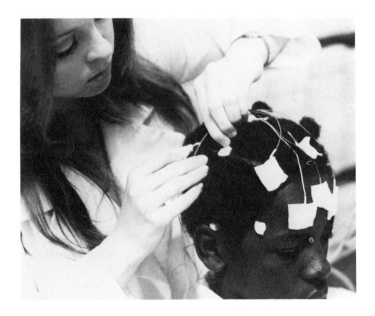

Figure 6-1
Electrodes are secured to the scalp before electroencephalography.

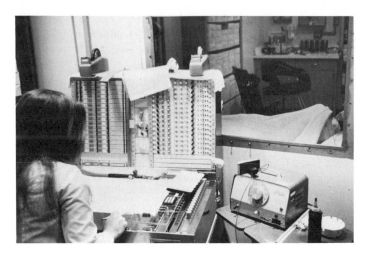

Figure 6-2
Electroencephalogram is recorded as the child lies comfortably in the
darkened adjacent room. A large picture window facilitates constant
visualization of the child.

stories. Smaller babies may be given a bottle. Readings are
taken while the child is awake and continued as he falls
asleep. Sleep EEGs are helpful because abnormal wave
forms not seen on the waking record may become visible.
Recordings taken while the child is hyperventilating may
also be helpful. Alkalosis resulting from hyperventilation
(30 to 40 respirations per minute for 3 minutes) accen-
tuates any abnormal brain wave activity that may be
present. External distractions should be kept to a mini-
mum during the test.

Preparation: The child's hair may be shampooed to remove oils that would interfere with electrode readings.
Glasses, hairpins, barrettes, or ribbons must be removed.
If a sleep EEG is performed, the child should be kept
awake for 8 to 10 hours before the study.

The purpose of the EEG should be explained to the

child and parents. Placement of the electrodes should be explained. The child may need reassurance that his head will not be shaved nor will his hair be cut. The EEG is not painful; electricity does not flow into the child, so he will not feel a shock. Upon first seeing the EEG equipment, some children are afraid of electrocution.

The child may experience the following during the EEG:

- Sixteen electrodes will be attached with paste to various places on his scalp. This will take approximately 15 minutes.

- He will be asked to lie quietly in a darkened room for a period of time and will probably go to sleep for a while.

- He may be asked to breathe as fast and as hard as he can for several minutes during the test.

- After the test, the electrodes will be removed and the paste will be washed from his hair.

Aftercare: The electrode paste should be washed from the child's hair. If the paste has dried, vigorous brushing often removes a great deal of it. Acetone may be used to remove dried paste, but this substance should be used with caution on infants' and young children's sensitive skin. Adequate ventilation is essential if acetone is used. Baby oil is sometimes helpful to soften dried paste. It is important to remove the electrode paste from the child's hair as soon as possible since large amounts of dried paste are extremely difficult to remove. The child should be encouraged to rest after an EEG.

Interpretation of Findings: The record is examined and interpreted according to the frequency, amplitude, and characteristics of the brain waves. The predominating frequencies of the EEG may be modified by many factors, for example, opening and closing of the eyes, state of consciousness, and drugs (9).

Spike discharges (abnormal, sharp, higher voltage wave-forms, often followed by a slow wave) are characteristic of epilepsy. Abnormalities that occur repeatedly and at regular intervals are called *periodic complexes.* These abnormalities may be generalized, focal (localized), or multifocal. Generalized slowing reveals a process affecting the entire brain and may indicate pressure that is causing problems in both hemispheres or some other generalized process such as toxic or metabolic encephalopathy, intracranial hemorrhage, or hypoxemia. A focal slowing reveals a process restricted to one area and may indicate a local disturbance causing destruction of brain tissue. Finally, a multifocal slowing reveals several areas of abnormality.

LUMBAR PUNCTURE

Lumbar puncture, or spinal tap, is an invasive procedure in which a hollow needle is inserted into the lumbar subarachnoid space of the spinal canal. Lumbar puncture, one of the simplest and most informative neurological diagnostic tests, may be performed to evaluate intracranial pressure, to obtain culture, sensitivity, cell count, sugar, and protein of cerebrospinal fluid, or to identify hemorrhage in the central nervous system.

Lumbar puncture may also be used for the administration of anesthetic or medication as part of another procedure (e.g., myelography, pneumoencephalography). Lumbar puncture is contraindicated in the presence of a space-occupying lesion that produces increased intracranial pressure (papilledema) or an untreated clotting defect.

Lumbar puncture is dangerous in the presence of increased intracranial pressure because the rapid reduction of pressure caused by removal of CSF can cause herniation of the brain structures (cerebellar tonsils) into the foramen magnum. This would put pressure on the medulla (e.g., the respiratory center) and could cause sudden death (1).

Premedication: None.

Diet: Usually no restriction necessary. If determination of CSF glucose is very important (suspected infection), the child may be kept NPO several hours before the lumbar puncture, since CSF glucose lags 1 to 2 hours behind serum glucose.

Consent: An authorization signed by the parent or guardian is advisable.

Time: 10 to 30 minutes, depending on the difficulty of placing the needle and the speed at which the CSF drips from the spinal canal.

Procedure: The child is restrained in the lateral recumbent position on the treatment room table (see Appendix A). For the infant the sitting position may be preferable (see "Restraint Necessary"). The skin is cleansed with iodine and alcohol and draped with sterile towels or a special drape. The physician wears sterile gloves and pays meticulous attention to sterile technique, since carelessness may result in a potentially fatal infection. Local anesthesia is accomplished by subcutaneous infiltration of 1% procaine. The spinal needle is then inserted between the third and fourth lumbar vertebrae. Since the spinal cord ends at the upper margin of the third lumbar vertebra in infants (and at or above L-1 in older children), puncture between the third and fourth lumbar vertebrae minimizes danger of injuring the spinal cord (1). Once the needle is in position, the stylet is removed and a stopcock and manometer are attached to measure the initial CSF pressure before any fluid is removed. In collecting the CSF specimens, the physician allows the fluid to drip into a series of three small sterile test tubes. One milliliter of fluid is collected in each of the tubes, which are then numbered and sent to the laboratory for examination. Closing pressure may be measured at the completion of CSF collection. Pressure measurements are meaningless in a struggling, crying patient, so the child must be encouraged to relax by reassurance and appropriate distraction. After the necessary specimens and pressure measurements are obtained, the needle is quickly withdrawn and pressure applied for several minutes with a sterile gauze. A Band-Aid is placed over the puncture site.

Preparation: The child should be told the reason for the procedure and that the doctor will take a small sample of spinal fluid from the lower spine. The child will be told to lie on his side with his legs pulled up close to his chin. It may be helpful to ask the child to try to touch his knees to his chin and to "curl up in a ball." He must lie still during the procedure. There will be someone to help him hold still, but he must understand the importance of cooperating. Sensations during the lumbar puncture will be:

- a cold feeling while the skin is being cleansed with an antiseptic solution
- a stinging or burning sensation for a few seconds while the local anesthetic is being injected
- a feeling of pressure when the spinal needle is inserted
- perhaps brief, sharp pains down his legs or hips (if the needle touches nerves that run to those areas) for a few moments.

The child should be reassured that the entire procedure will last only a few minutes and that only a few drops of spinal fluid will be removed.

After the lumbar puncture, the child must stay flat in bed until he is rested. He will be encouraged to drink liquids during that time.

Restraint Necessary: The success of this procedure depends largely on the skill with which the child is restrained.

The child is positioned on his side with knees flexed on the abdomen and head flexed on the chest, thereby separating the vertebrae and increasing the space between them. The sitting position is often used in small infants who have low CSF pressure. It is essential to provide constant verbal support during the procedure. The child should be observed for tolerance to the procedure. Respiratory status, in particular, must be monitored closely.

Aftercare: The child should be kept flat in bed, but not necessarily on his back, until rested. Although postpuncture headache is not as common in children as in adults, it may be relieved by analgesics and is often minimized by liberal fluid intake and bedrest in the horizontal position. Postpuncture headache is most likely to occur when large amounts of CSF have been removed rapidly or when leakage from the spinal canal into the subarachnoid space has occurred (10).

The child should be observed for pain or hematoma at the puncture site, leakage of CSF, difficulty in voiding, or any change in neurological status. Dangerous trends that should be reported immediately include pupillary changes, especially dilation of one or both pupils, decreased level of consciousness, loss or decline of motor ability or bowel and bladder function, and marked change in vital signs, especially a rise in blood pressure, lowered pulse, or respiratory difficulty (11).

Normal Values: See Appendix B-6.

MYELOGRAPHY

Myelography is an invasive procedure in which the spinal cord and vertebral canal are visualized radiographically following injection of a contrast medium into the lumbar or cisternal subarachnoid space. Myelography is useful in identifying tumors, masses, fractures, foreign bodies, dislocations, or interference in the flow of CSF.

Premedication: A sedative with atropine may be administered 20 to 30 minutes before the procedure.

Diet: The child is kept NPO for 6 to 8 hours before the study to prevent aspiration from nausea and vomiting that may result from the lumbar or cisternal puncture or the tilting of the table.

Consent: An authorization signed by the parent or guardian is necessary.

Time: Approximately 2 hours.

Procedure: A lumbar puncture is performed (see lumbar puncture) with the child in a lateral, prone, or sitting position on the tilting x-ray table. Placement of the needle is checked fluoroscopically. A small amount of CSF is allowed to drip out and is replaced by a positive contrast agent (such as Pantopaque or metrizamide) or a negative contrast agent (air). The child is tilted to various angles on the x-ray table and the flow of contrast medium up and down the spinal canal is observed fluoroscopically. X-ray films are taken with the child in various positions. He should be securely restrained to prevent slipping on the tilting x-ray table. When the appropriate films have been taken, the table is tilted to cause the contrast medium to collect around the puncture needle. If insoluble contrast medium such as Pantopaque was used, it is removed as completely as possible by allowing it to drip out through the needle or with gentle suction with a syringe. Water soluble contrast materials such as metrizamide are resorbed spontaneously. The needle is withdrawn, pressure applied for a few minutes, and a Band-Aid is placed over the site.

Preparation: The child should be checked for any allergy to iodine or iodine products to prevent anaphylaxis. The procedure should be explained simply and clearly to the parents and child. They should be prepared for the period of time the child is NPO and for the sedative. A baseline record of vital signs and neurological status should be obtained before the child is premedicated. All jewelry, safety pins, and other metal items should be removed to prevent extraneous shadows from appearing on the x-ray films. The child must understand the importance of holding still during the procedure.

The child will experience the following sensations:

- drowsiness and dryness of the mouth from the premedication
- a stinging sensation in the back (lumbar puncture) or base of skull (cisternal puncture) while the puncture site is being anesthetized with procaine
- a feeling of pressure when the lumbar puncture needle is inserted
- motion when the tilting x-ray table changes positions
- radiating, stabbing, sharp pain in the back for a few minutes while the contrast material is being removed.

Restraint Necessary: The child must understand the importance of remaining still during the procedure. He may be restrained as for a lumbar puncture (see "Lumbar Puncture") during puncture and instillation of the contrast medium. After that, calm reassurance and snug support on the tilting table are usually sufficient.

Aftercare: If the contrast medium has been removed completely or a water soluble compound was used, the child may remain flat in bed for a few hours and then resume normal activities. If the insoluble material has not been removed, the child's head must be kept elevated above the level of the spine to prevent irritative chemical meningitis. The child should be observed for signs of meningeal irritation.

After air myelography, the child must be kept in a head-down position for 48 hours to prevent the air from entering the intracranial subarachnoid space.

The child should be observed for fever or any alterations of intracranial pressure for 24 to 48 hours. Fluids should be encouraged to assist in replacement of CSF, rehydration, and removal of the contrast material through the urine.

PNEUMOENCEPHALOGRAPHY

Pneumoencephalography is an invasive procedure in which air is injected into the subarachnoid space and ventricular system from a lumbar or cisternal site*. Because air is radiolucent compared to cerebral soft tissues and bone, the size, shape, symmetry, and position of the ventricular system and subarachnoid spaces may be visualized radiographically. Such information is valuable in defining anatomy along the brain stem and base of the skull, areas not well seen with the CAT scan.

Premedication: Since pneumoencephalography is usually performed under general anesthesia, a preoperative sedative may be given before the procedure. Demerol may potentiate hypotension and should not be used before pneumoencephalography (12).

---

*Pneumoencephalography has largely replaced ventriculography, the injection of air directly into the ventricles through the open sutures of the infant or through trephine holes in the older child. However, when there is a possibility of an expanding lesion or of increased intracranial pressure, ventriculography is the procedure of choice because of lessened risk of brain stem herniation (12).

Diet: The child should be NPO for 6 to 8 hours before the study to prevent vomiting and possible aspiration of gastric contents.

Consent: An authorization signed by the parent or guardian is necessary.

Time: 2 to 4 hours.

Procedure: General anesthesia is induced and the child is prepped the same as for a lumbar puncture or cisternal puncture. (Usually the lumbar route is used for pneumoencephalograms. The cisternal route is more hazardous from the standpoint of puncture technique.) With the child in a sitting position, a lumbar puncture is performed. Free flow of CSF is established and air is injected in 5 to 10 cc increments. Since air is lighter than CSF, it rises into the ventricular system. Injection of air is continued until 20 to 30 cc of air have been injected and adequate filling of the ventricular system has been obtained. At the end of the air injections, several milliliters of CSF are removed for biochemical and cytological examination. The needle is then withdrawn and x-ray films are taken. The child's position is rotated from erect to brow-up and brow-down positions to allow air to flow from one part of the cerebral ventricular system to another. Once all the necessary views have been taken, the child is placed in a supine position and taken to the recovery room. There he is allowed to awaken from the general anesthesia and is returned to his room when fully awake.

Preparation: The child's hair should be clean and free of braids or matting that might produce extraneous shadows on the x-ray films. Hairpins, necklaces, or other metal objects should be removed. Baseline vital signs and neurological vital signs should be checked and recorded immediately before the procedure. These measurements are essential in interpreting postprocedure measurements.

The purpose of the test should be explained simply and clearly to the child and parents. The child should be prepared for general anesthesia and understand that he may have a headache when he wakes up. The headache is normal and will disappear within a day or so. The child will be given medication to lessen the discomfort.

The child should be told that his vital signs and neuro-vital signs (shining a light in his eyes, asking him to squeeze the nurse's hand, etc.) will be checked frequently and that such frequent monitoring does not mean something is wrong.

Aftercare: The child should remain flat in bed for 24 hours. Neurovital signs and vital signs are checked every 30 minutes for 2 hours, then every 1 to 2 hours as appropriate and compared with baseline measurements.

Headache, nausea, vomiting, irritability, and fever are the most common aftereffects and should receive symptomatic treatment. No analgesics containing antipyretics (for example, aspirin, Tylenol, Empirin #3) should be given, since they mask the symptoms of infection. Comfort measures are important and the room should be kept semidark and quiet since the child will have increased irritability to stimuli following the test. If not contraindicated, fluids should be encouraged to help replenish CSF.

SUBDURAL TAP

A subdural tap or ventricular tap is an invasive procedure performed to identify subdural effusions, subdural or ventricular hemorrhage, or bacteria in the subdural or ventricular spaces. A specimen of CSF for culture may be obtained, medication instilled, or intracranial pressure relieved during the subdural tap (13). This procedure is generally restricted to infants or children whose sutures are still open.

Premedication: If the subdural tap is to be performed during craniotomy, a preoperative sedative will be given before the procedure. Otherwise, no premedication is needed.

Diet: If the tap is to be performed during craniotomy, the child should be NPO for at least 4 to 6 hours before surgery. Otherwise, no dietary restrictions are necessary.

Consent: An authorization signed by the parent or guardian is necessary.

Time: 20 to 30 minutes. If performed during craniotomy, time is extremely variable.

Procedure: The anterior two-thirds of the scalp is shaved and strict aseptic technique observed throughout the procedure. A mummy restraint is applied and the head held securely. The operative area is carefully cleansed with an iodine solution and then alcohol. A sterile towel is placed under the child's head and another is draped across the posterior half of the skull. Wearing sterile gloves, the physician identifies the puncture site, either at the junction of the anterior fontanel and coronal suture, or, if the fontanel is small, a few millimeters away from the fontanel in the suture line. The area is anesthetized with procaine. A short lumbar puncture needle is then introduced. Once the scalp and skull are penetrated, the stylet is removed and fluid, if present, is allowed to drain. If fluid is not encountered, the needle is advanced approximately 0.5 to 1.0 cm until the dura mater has been punctured. Tubes of fluid are labeled and numbered in the order they are collected. Usually, subdural taps are performed bilaterally. The needle is changed before the second tap, since tiny clots or serum may cling to the inside of the needle used for the initial puncture. No more than 20 to 25 ml of fluid should be removed at one time, since removal of 30 ml or more may result in sudden intracranial decompression and shock. When collection is completed, the needle is withdrawn and a sterile dressing or collodion applied.

The child should be closely observed for tolerance throughout the procedure.

Preparation: The procedure should be explained simply and clearly to the parents of the child. The anterior two-thirds of the scalp will be shaved clean of hair, so the parents should be made aware of this before the consent form is signed. The child will experience the following sensations during the procedure:

- firm restraint of head and entire body during the procedure
- a stinging sensation on the top of the head as local anesthetic is injected
- a feeling of pressure as the subdural needle is inserted.

Restraint Necessary: It is imperative that the child be completely immobilized during a subdural tap. He should be placed on his back with his head facing forward. A mummy restraint is effective for immobilizing the body while an assistant holds the head firmly with one hand on either side of the face.

Aftercare: The child should be kept flat in bed for 24 hours and observed for changes in intracranial pressure or leakage of fluid from the puncture site. Vital signs should be monitored frequently (every 30 minutes) until stable.

REFERENCES

1. Luckmann J, Sorensen KC: *Medical-Surgical Nursing.* Philadelphia, W B Saunders Co, 1974.
2. Donohoe KM, Blount M, Kinney AB: Cerebral Circulation and Cerebral Angiography. *Nurs Clin North Am* 9(4):623, 1974.

3. Bhave DG, Kelsey CA, Burstein J, et al: Scattered Radiation Doses to Infants and Children During EMI Head Scans. *Radiology* 124(3):379, 1977.
4. Bronzino JD: *Technology for Patient Care.* St Louis, C V Mosby Co, 1977.
5. Pinto ES, Becker MH: Computed Tomography in Pediatric Diagnosis. *Am J Dis Child* 131(5):583, 1977.
6. Backman DS, Hughes FJ, Freeman JM: Computerized Axial Tomography in Neurologic Disorders of Children. *Pediatrics* 59:352, 1977.
7. McCullough DC, Kufta C, Axelbaum SP: Computerized Axial Tomography in Clinical Pediatrics. *Pediatrics* 59(2):173, 1977.
8. Conway BL: *Pediatric Neurologic Nursing.* St Louis, C V Mosby Co, 1977.
9. Lewis DV, Freeman JL: The Electroencephalogram in Pediatric Practice. *Pediatrics* 60(3):325, 1977.
10. Kempe CH, Silver HK, Obrien, D: *Current Pediatric Diagnosis and Treatment.* Los Altos, Ca, Lange Medical Publications, 1974.
11. Blount M, Kinney AB, Donohoe KM: Obtaining and Analyzing Cerebrospinal Fluid. *Nurs Clin North Am* 9(4):593, 1974.
12. Kinney AB, Blount M, Donohoe KM: Cerebrospinal Fluid Circulation and Encephalography. *Nurs Clin North Am* 9(4):611, 1974.
13. Scipien GM, Barnard MU, Howe J et al: *Comprehensive Pediatric Nursing.* New York, McGraw-Hill Book Co, 1975.

BIBLIOGRAPHY

Ambrose J: Computerized X-ray Scanning of the Brain. *J Neurosurg* 40:679, 1974.

Anderson RE, Osborn AG: Efficacy of Simple Sedation for Pediatric Computer Tomography. *Radiology* 124(3):739, 1977.

Bhave DG, Kelsey CA, Burstein J et al: Scattered Radiation Doses to Infants and Children During EMI Head Scans. *Radiology* 124(3):379, 1977.

Blount M, Kinney AB, Donohoe KM: Obtaining and Analyzing Cerebrospinal Fluid. *Nurs Clin North Am* 9(4):593, 1974.

Bronzino JD: *Technology for Patient Care.* St Louis, C V Mosby Co, 1977.

Byrd SE, Harwood-Nash DC, Barry JF, et al: Coronal Computed Tomography of the Skull and Brain in Infants and Children. *Radiology* 124(3):705, 1977.

Conway BL: *Pediatric Neurologic Nursing.* St Louis, C V Mosby Co, 1977.

Day RE, Thomson JL, Schutt WH: Computerized Axial Tomography and Acute Neurological Problems of Childhood. *Arch Dis Child* 53(1):2, 1978.

Donohoe KM, Blount M, Kinney AB: Cerebral Circulation and Cerebral Angiography. *Nurs Clin North Am* 9(4):623, 1974.

Gomez, MR, Reese DF: Computed Tomography of the Head in Infants and Children. *Pediatr Clin North Am* 23(3):473, 1976.

Kinney AB, Blount M, Donohoe KM: Cerebrospinal Fluid Circulation and Encephalography. *Nurs Clin North Am* 9(4):611, 1971.

Knight DR, LePortz MT, Harper JR: Natural Sleep as an Aid to Electroencephalographic Diagnosis in Young Children. *Dev Med Child Neurol* 19(4):503, 1977.

Lewis DV, Freeman JM: The Electroencephalogram in Pediatric Practice. *Pediatrics* 60(3):324, 1977.

Luckman J, Sorensen KC: *Medical Surgical Nursing.* Philadelphia, W B Saunders Co, 1974.

Mandrillo MP: Brain Scanning. *Nurs Clin North Am* 9(4):633, 1974.

Nelson, WE, Vaughan VC, McKay RF: *Textbook of Pediatrics,* ed 10. Philadelphia, W B Saunders Co, 1975.

Pinto ES, Becker MH: Computed Tomography in Pediatric Diagnosis. *Am J Dis Child* 131(5):583, 1977.

7

Gastrointestinal Diagnostic Procedures

BARIUM ENEMA

A barium enema is an invasive radiologic procedure used to visualize the colon.

Premedication: None.

Diet: Many radiology departments require a low residue supper and NPO after midnight before the procedure. Foods in a low residue diet include tender meats, eggs, bread and cereals without roughage or bulk, clear soups, pureed bland vegetables and fruits, soft desserts, and boiled milk.

Time: 35 to 45 minutes.

Procedure: The child is placed on the x-ray table and the rectal catheter is inserted. Foley or other types of balloon catheters should be used cautiously since they may obscure the rectal area and damage the rectal mucosa (1). The disposable enema tip may be secured by taping the buttocks firmly together. The barium is allowed to flow into the colon by gravity from a height of 18 inches above the hips. A towel or some absorbent material should be placed beneath the child's buttocks. The radiologist watches the advancing column of barium on the fluoroscopic screen while the patient is rotated to different positions. The flow of barium is stopped each time a spot film is taken. Some form of abdominal compression may be applied intermittently during the examination to separate overlapping loops of bowel. After the x-ray films are taken, the patient may be helped to the bathroom to expel the barium. If the child is not bowel trained, the barium may be removed by lowering the enema reservoir and allowing the barium to be siphoned back into the container. Then, with a towel under the infant's buttocks, the tube is withdrawn. Postevacuation films are usually obtained. A 24-hour delayed film will demonstrate the position of the cecum.

Air contrast studies are not commonly utilized in children but may be of value in detecting polyps. After evacuation of the barium, the bowel is distended with air and x-rays are taken. The thin film of barium adhering to the mucosa permits visualization of minute lesions.

Preparation: Adequate cleansing of the colon is necessary to promote visualization. In the examination for suspected polyps, thorough cleansing is imperative. Bowel preparation may be accomplished in children younger than 5 years with two or three saline cleansing enemas (40 ml/kg body weight) before the examination. Children 5 years and older may be prepared with one ounce of castor oil at 4:00 PM the day before and cleansing enemas before the examination. The castor oil may be taken more readily if mixed with a sweet carbonated beverage or fruit juice. Enemas are of value not only in cleansing the colon but also for emotional preparation. If the child is told that this is similar to the x-ray examination, his anxiety may be decreased at the time of fluoroscopy.

If the barium enema is being done for evaluation of constipation, megacolon, or intussusception, no cathartics or enemas should be given. If the barium enema is being administered through a colostomy, no castor oil is given, but the morning irrigation is more vigorous than usual and the diet consists of clear liquids for a day before the examination.

The child should be prepared for the enemas as well as for the trip to the x ray room, positioning on the x-ray table, and insertion of the rectal tube. The enema tubing will be secured to the buttocks with tape. The child will experience a feeling of fullness when the barium is instilled and pressure when compression is applied to the abdomen. The child will be placed in different positions as several x-ray films are taken.

Barium enema must be performed before upper GI studies if a possibility of colon obstruction exists to prevent inspissation of barium in the colon proximal to the obstruction. Most institutions routinely perform the barium enema first to avoid this complication. Barium enema must be performed after excretory pyelography or oral cholecystography. Sigmoidoscopy should be done at least 24 hours before a barium enema since the introduction of air during sigmoidoscopy, increased spasm of the colon, and the secretion of mucus result in an unsatisfactory barium enema (1). If biopsy was performed with sigmoidoscopy, there should be a delay of at least 7 days to decrease the possibility of perforation at the site of biopsy.

Restraint Necessary: The child must remain still while the x-ray films are being taken. Gentle restraint by lead-aproned personnel will accomplish this.

Aftercare: Cleansing enemas and castor oil must be administered to rid the colon of barium, which could cause an impaction. Fluids should be encouraged to promote rehydration.

COLONOSCOPY

Colonoscopy is an invasive procedure that provides direct visualization of the colon as far as the ileocecal junction. The flexible fiberoptic colonoscope makes a larger portion of the colon accessible for examination or polyp removal than the traditional sigmoidoscope. The colonoscope operates like other flexible endoscopes (see "Upper GI Endoscopy").

Premedication: Colonoscopy may be performed under general anesthesia (2,3,5) or with sedation alone (4,6,7,-8,9). If general anesthesia is used, the child will receive a routine preoperative medication approximately 1 hour before the procedure. In the older child and adolescent, sedation may be deemed adequate and can be achieved with an IM narcotic and atropine 1 hour before the examination. If polyp removal is anticipated, additional sedation may be provided with IV diazepam (Valium) at the time of the examination. Some physicians prefer that their patients be awake to inform them of the onset of pain, a possible warning sign of impending perforation or of a false passage of the colonoscope into a diverticular fold (6).

Diet: The child is given a clear liquid diet 24 hours before the procedure.

Consent: An authorization signed by the parent or guardian is necessary.

Time: 30 minutes.

Procedure: The child is placed in a left lateral recumbent position on the examination table. The anal canal and the tip of the colonoscope are well lubricated with a water-soluble lubricant. The tip is introduced gently through the anal canal and the instrument is passed under direct visualization as far as possible. The location of the tip may be checked by fluoroscopy, but the use of fluoroscopy is usually limited since radiation damages the fiber glass bundles, gradually producing a yellowing effect. During the examination the child may feel some gas pains due to the air insufflation that opens the lumen of the colon for better visualization. The entire intestinal mucosa is carefully inspected as the colonoscope is slowly withdrawn. Photographs may be taken, superficial biopsy specimens excised, and lesions brushed for cytology. Polyps and tumors may also be excised by the experienced endoscopist.

Preparation: Cleansing of the bowel is essential for adequate visualization of the colon. The bowel is prepared with two or three warm isotonic saline enemas until clear (40 ml/kg body weight) the day before and a 60-ml Fleet enema at least 3 hours before the examination. The time interval between the last enema and examination is necessary to avoid retention of excess fluid in the colon (8). The administration of cathartics is controversial; it has been noted that both castor oil and magnesium sulfate can cause mucosal changes in the colon (hyperemia, edema, congestion of the vascular networks) simulating pathologic conditions (6). Platelet count and prothrombin time should be checked in anticipation of possible biopsy or polypectomy.

The child should be prepared for the enemas with an explanation of their purpose. A simple description of the colonoscopy should be provided. It is most helpful for the child to see the flexible scope before the examination, to touch it, and look through it. This activity stimulates questions about the procedure and helps dispel anxiety for the child awaiting colonoscopy. The child may experience a cramping sensation when the bowel is insufflated with air and some discomfort due to the presence of the instrument in the colon. The child should be told it is important for him to remain still during the examination and to tell the examiner if he feels pain. An understanding nurse with a matter of fact attitude will do much to decrease the child's embarrassment.

If the examination is to be performed under general anesthesia, the child should be told in simple terms what will happen to him while he is asleep, where he will wake up, and when he will be able to resume normal diet and activity.

Restraint Necessary: If the procedure is not performed

under general anesthesia, immobilization may be accomplished with adequate sedation and explanation. The calm reassurance of the nurse during the procedure is helpful in obtaining a relaxed abdomen and a cooperative patient.

Aftercare: If general anesthesia was used, the child is observed in the recovery room until fully awake. Otherwise, the child is returned to his room on a stretcher. Vital signs should be checked and side rails raised until effects of the medication have worn off.

If polyps were excised, the child should be on a low-residue diet for one week. The child should be observed for signs of bleeding if polyps were removed or a biopsy specimen obtained.

INTRAVENOUS CHOLANGIOGRAPHY

Intravenous cholangiography, an invasive radiologic procedure used to visualize the biliary duct system, has limited usefulness in the pediatric age group and is not without risk (anaphylaxis). Usually IV cholangiography is preceded by oral cholangiography.

Premedication: None.

Diet: The evening before the procedure the child should be given a light nonfat meal and nothing by mouth after midnight.

Consent: An authorization signed by the parent or guardian is necessary.

Time: 2 to 4 hours.

Procedure: The child is placed in a supine position on the x-ray table with his right side elevated and a scout film is taken before the injection of the contrast material. An IV is started and the contrast material, Cholografin meglumine (meglumine iodipamide injection USP) is infused within 10 to 15 minutes. X-ray films are then taken at 15-minute intervals until the desired information is obtained. X-rays may be taken up to 4 hours after the contrast material is injected, allowing the gallbladder to fill with dye and excrete it into the intestine. Tomographic cuts* may be obtained, particularly when extraneous shadows do not permit adequate visualization" (10).

The child should be observed for common side effects of Cholografin such as nausea, vomiting, hypotension, urticaria, and flushing. More severe reactions to the contrast material (anaphylaxis) may occur but are infrequent.

Preparation: The child should be checked for allergy to seafood or iodine to prevent anaphylaxis.

Some radiology departments request that the child's bowel be cleared with a cathartic and/or enemas to promote visualization. The child should be prepared for this, for the period of time he will be NPO, for pain during venipuncture, and for the long wait between x-ray films. Intravenous cholangiography must precede any barium study.

---

*Tomograms, laminagrams, planigrams, or body section roetgenograms: By adjusting the x-ray equipment so that there is a simultaneous movement of the x-ray tube and the film in opposite directions about a specific plane, all structures are blurred out, leaving only a selected layer of an organ in clear view. Films obtained in this manner are often called tomographic cuts. The two x-ray tubes that make up tomographic equipment are suspended over the x-ray table. When the cuts are being made, these swing rapidly and abruptly in converging and then in diverging paths above the patient. This rapid swooping may frighten the patient if he is not forewarned (11).

Restraint Necessary: The child must remain completely still while x-ray films are being taken. If tomographic cuts are taken, this may be a considerable length of time. Foam wedges may help the child maintain his position.

Aftercare: No physical aftercare required unless an untoward reaction to the contrast material occurs.

Interpretation: Cystic dilatation and tumors of the bile ducts may be detected by IV cholangiography. Of course, this test is of no value in the jaundiced patient since the dye would not be sufficiently metabolized in the liver and concentrated in the gallbladder for visualization.

IONTOPHORETIC SWEAT TEST

The iontophoretic sweat test, pilocarpine iontophoresis, is a noninvasive procedure that measures sweat electrolyte concentration. A small electric current carries pilocarpine into the skin and stimulates sweat glands locally. This simple test, the diagnostic procedure of choice for cystic fibrosis, is about 98% reliable in establishing the diagnosis.

Premedication: None.

Diet: No special diet necessary.

Time: 45 minutes.

Procedure: The area to be iontophoresed (forearm in older children, scapula or thigh in infants) is washed with distilled water and dried. A 2 × 2 inch gauze, moistened with 2 ml of 0.5% pilocarpine nitrate solution, is placed on the forearm. The positive copper electrode is positioned on the gauze so that it is not in contact with the skin and is secured with a rubber strap (Fig. 7-1). The negative copper electrode is placed elsewhere on the arm on top of gauze soaked in saline. The two electrodes are firmly attached with rubber straps similar to the kind used for electrocardiography. The lead wires are then connected, the power supply switched on, and the current slowly increased to 0.5 mamp in 15 to 20 seconds. Iontophoresis is continued for 5 minutes. If the patient complains of a tingling sensation, pressing firmly on the offending electrode is helpful.

After completion of iontophoresis the electrodes are removed, the gauze with the pilocarpine is discarded and the skin under the positive electrode is washed with distilled water and dried. A thin pad of gauze is removed with forceps from the bottle in which it was previously weighed and placed over the site of sweating (positive electrode). The gauze is then covered with a square of Parafilm and sealed at the edges with waterproof tape to

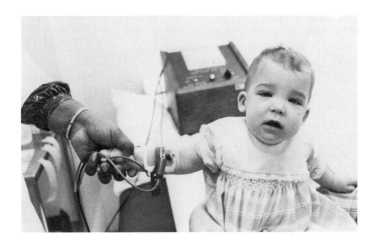

Figure 7-1
Pilocarpine iontophoresis. Note the electrode secured to the forearm on top of a saline-soaked gauze. Power supply unit is in the background.

prevent evaporation. After 30 minutes the gauze is removed with forceps and reweighed in the same bottle. The bottle should be tightly capped immediately to prevent evaporation. The difference in weights represents the amount of sweat collected, assuming that 1 ml of sweat weights 1 gr. A 50-mg sample must be obtained for a reliable result.

Preparation: No physical preparation is needed. The child and parents will need support when they face the implications of a positive diagnosis. An explanation should be given in simple terms of what is going to be done and why. The child should be reassured that the test is painless. A tingling sensation may be experienced for a few seconds.

Aftercare: No physical aftercare is necessary.

Normal Values:

Normal children	40 mEq/L or less
Cystic fibrosis patients	60–100 mEq/L or more
Adults	80 mEq/L or less

A few children suspected of having cystic fibrosis may fall into a borderline range of 50 to 70 mEq/L. These children require repeated sweat tests and continued clinical observation.

LIVER BIOPSY

Liver biopsy is an invasive procedure by which a sample of liver tissue is obtained for microscopic examination. Liver biopsy may be helpful in patients with prolonged jaundice, biliary atresia, suspected liver disease, portal hypertension, neoplasms of the liver, or Reye's syndrome.

Premedication: The child must be adequately sedated.

An IM narcotic is administered 1 hour before the procedure.

Diet: The child is kept NPO for at least 4 hours before the procedure.

Consent: An authorization signed by the parent or guardian is necessary.

Time: 10 minutes.

Procedure: The child is placed in a supine position with his arms restrained at his sides. The biopsy site is selected by percussion, and the area is cleansed with an antiseptic solution and draped. The skin, subcutaneous tissues, and muscles are infiltrated with local anesthestic. Some physicians also infiltrate the liver capsule. A very small skin incision is made at the biopsy site and a trocar is passed through the intercostal muscles to form a tract for the biopsy needle (Fig. 7-2). Then the biopsy needle*, attached to a syringe, is inserted through the incision and the tract left by the trocar until the liver is encountered. A core of liver tissue is aspirated and the needle removed. The needle is in the liver less than 1 second.

Pressure is placed on the biopsy site for 5 to 10 minutes and a dressing is firmly applied.

Preparation: The child's hematocrit and blood count are checked and partial thromboplastin time (PTT), prothrombin time, platelet count, and bleeding time are also evaluated. Liver biopsy is contraindicated in the presence of any bleeding tendency. The child's blood is typed, cross-matched, and held on call.

---

*Several types of biopsy needles are used. The most popular are the Vim-Silverman, the Roth-Turkel, and the Menghini. The Menghini needle provides a more rapid and effective means of removing tissue than the other types.

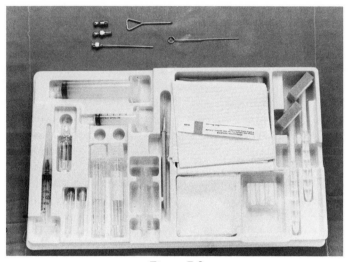

Figure 7-2
Liver biopsy tray with liver biopsy needle.

The child should be prepared for the IM injection and the drowsy feeling following it. He should also be told that he will feel a cold sensation when the skin is cleansed with an antiseptic solution, stinging when the skin over the liver is infiltrated with local anesthetic, and pressure when the biopsy needle is inserted. The child may have pain at the puncture site for a few hours after the procedure that will be relieved with analgesics. It is important for the child to understand the necessity of remaining still during the biopsy. He will be asked to hold his breath for a few seconds when the needle is inserted. A practice session may be helpful. He should also be assured that someone will be with him to help him hold still.

After the biopsy the child must stay in bed on his right side for several hours. He cannot eat or drink during this time and nurses will be checking him very often.

Restraint Necessary: Immobilization is imperative for a safe procedure. Infants may be restrained on a circumcision board. Older children are placed in a supine position with the arms restrained at the sides or above the head. The older child will be asked to hold his breath when the needle is inserted. Manual immobilization of the abdomen is helpful in infants and small children.

Aftercare: The child should be kept NPO and on his right side in bed for several hours. Vital signs should be checked frequently to monitor for bleeding and resultant shock (every 15 minutes for 1 hour, every 30 minutes for 1 hour, and then, every hour for 4 hours). Hematocrit may also be checked every 4 hours until stabilized.

Infrequent complications of liver biopsy include local pain and infection, bile peritonitis, intrahepatic hematoma, and hemorrhage. Complications may be minimized by proper preparation, by restraint, and by attention to aftercare.

ORAL CHOLECYSTOGRAPHY

Oral cholecystography is a noninvasive radiologic procedure used to visualize the gallbladder and sometimes the cystic and common bile ducts. Its greatest value is in showing stones and gallbladder disease, both of which are uncommon, but may be seen occasionally, in the pediatric age group.

Premedication: Oral radiopaque tablets, iopanoic acid (Telepaque), are given on the evening before the test, during or after a light, nonfat meal. Patients with cystic fibrosis should receive an extra dose of pancreatic enzyme supplements with the Telepaque as well as extra pancreatic enzymes 36 and 12 hours before the x-ray examination.

Diet: The child is given a light, nonfat meal the evening

before the examination and is kept NPO until the films are taken. After the x-ray examination, the child may receive either a fatty meal or a commercially available cholecystagogue if additional x-ray films for evidence of gallbladder contraction are needed.

Time: 30 to 45 minutes. Much of this time will be spent waiting between films while they are being developed and examined.

Procedure: Telepaque is administered in the evening with a fat-free meal and multiple films are taken the next morning. Occasionally, films that show gallbladder contraction may be desired. In such cases a fatty meal or a commercially available cholecystagogue will be given and then another film taken.

If the gallbladder is not visible, the dose of Telepaque is repeated and films are taken again in 6 to 8 hours.

Preparation: Plain abdominal scout films are taken before the radiopaque medium is given. Any allergies, especially to seafood or iodine, should be ascertained. Telepaque tablets are then administered with small amounts of water. The child should be observed for common side effects such as nausea and vomiting, which would alter the drug uptake. Some diarrhea may be expected, but this is usually mild and is helpful in clearing the intestinal tract and promoting visualization of the gallbladder. The evening meal should be fat-free. Appropriate foods would include fruit, bread or toast with jelly, juice, lean meat, and vegetables. No milk or butter may be used in this meal since fats stimulate the gallbladder, which must be relaxed in order to concentrate the contrast media.

The child should be prepared for the period of time he will be NPO. He should be told that he may have a considerable waiting period between x-ray films.

Aftercare: No physical aftercare is necessary.

Interpretation of Findings: Significant findings are the presence of gallstones, nonfunctioning gallbladder, and abnormal contraction. In children with liver disease, non-visualization of the gallbladder may occur because the contrast media is not excreted. If gallbladder disease is present, nonvisualization may occur because the media cannot be concentrated, a gallbladder lumen is absent, or a duct is obstructed.

This test is not successful in children with jaundice or biliary atresia. In the presence of liver disease, the patient is not able to metabolize and concentrate the dye in the gallbladder.

PERCUTANEOUS TRANSHEPATIC CHOLANGIOGRAPHY

Percutaneous transhepatic cholangiography is an invasive radiologic procedure used to visualize the hepatobiliary system. The major advantages of this type of cholangiography are that it may be used in jaundiced patients to differentiate between obstructive and nonobstructive (hepatocellular) jaundice and that it can better outline lesions in obstructive jaundice than is possible with operative cholangiography. If an obstruction is revealed, surgery is scheduled to follow within 6 hours after the procedure.

Premedication: Some physicians recommend that prophylactic antibiotics be given for two days before the procedure. The child is premedicated with meperidine (Demerol) and phenobarbitol 1 hour before the procedure.

Diet: The child is kept NPO for 8 to 12 hours before the procedure.

Consent: An authorization signed by the parent or guardian is necessary.

Time: 35 minutes to 2 hours if delayed films are needed. The patient may go directly to surgery following the procedure.

Procedure: An IV may be started in a peripheral vein as a precautionary measure to treat complications. The child is placed in a supine position on the fluoroscopy table and the skin over the right lower chest and upper abdomen is cleansed with an antiseptic solution and draped. The area to be injected is infiltrated with a local anesthetic down to and including the peritoneum. Various puncture sites are used. Many physicians prefer introducing the needle through the anterior abdominal wall two fingerbreadths below the right costal arch. Lateral or dorsal puncture sites are also used. To puncture the liver, either a catheter and needle assembly or a Chiba needle may be used. Using fluoroscopic visualization, the needle is introduced into the liver. If the child is old enough, he is instructed to hold his breath when the needle enters the liver. The needle connected to a syringe containing contrast material is slowly withdrawn until bile is aspirated, indicating that a duct has been entered. If a bile duct is not entered, the needle is inserted and withdrawn until bile appears in the syringe. In obstructive jaundice, the bile ducts are generally enlarged and easily located. Failure to enter a duct may indicate hepatocellular disease. The biliary system is then slowly and gently emptied and samples are sent to the laboratory for bacteriologic and cytologic studies. After bile has been aspirated, the contrast material is injected and the needle withdrawn. X-ray films are then taken in different positions. Delayed films may be taken 15 minutes to 2 hours after injection to provide information about the emptying of the biliary system. A needle biopsy of the liver may be done if attempts to enter a bile duct are unsuccessful.

If an obstructive lesion is revealed, surgery is usually performed within a few hours after the procedure.

Preparation: Blood clotting should be normal (prothrombin time within 3 seconds of the control). Broad spectrum antibiotics may be administered for two days before the procedure to prevent bile peritonitis. Gram-negative organisms frequently have been cultured from bile of patients with obstructive jaundice. The child should be checked for any allergy to iodine or iodine products. This procedure is contraindicated in the presence of a bleeding tendency, sensitivity to iodine, high fever or continuous fever around 38°C, extreme jaundice, ascites, moderate to severe anemia, and biliary tract infections (12,13).

The child should be prepared for the injection of the premedication and the drowsy feeling following it. Sensations the child will experience include pain during venipuncture if an IV is to be started, a cold feeling when the skin is cleansed with an antiseptic solution, and a stinging sensation when a local anesthetic is injected. The child must be helped to understand the importance of holding still during the remainder of the procedure. He should be told that he will be asked to hold his breath for a few seconds while the special needle is inserted. Practice sessions of breath holding may be helpful. The child will experience a feeling of pressure when the needle is inserted into the liver and moderate to severe pain for a few seconds while contrast media is being injected. The child may also have some degree of pain for a few hours after the procedure. He may be taken to surgery immediately after this procedure and should be prepared accordingly.

Restraint Necessary: To prevent hemorrhage, the child must remain completely motionless when the needle enters the liver. If he is old enough, he should also hold his breath for two to three seconds while the puncture is being done. The child must also be immobilized while the x-ray films are being taken. Adequate sedation is essential.

Aftercare: If an obstructive lesion is found, the child will be taken to surgery within a few hours. If surgery is not indicated, the child should be closely observed for hemorrhage due to a puncture of a blood vessel or a laceration of the liver. Bile peritonitis due to leakage of bile into the peritoneal cavity is another serious complication. Pain sometimes persists 3 or 4 hours after cholangiography and may be alleviated with analgesics. The child's vital signs (temperature, pulse, respiration, and blood pressure) should be checked frequently (every 15 minutes for 2 hours, every ½ hour for 2 hours, every hour for 4 hours, and then once every 3 hours). Septicemia and tension pneumothorax have been reported infrequently (14). Some physicians recommend that antibiotics be administered for three days after the procedure.

RECTOSIGMOIDOSCOPY

Rectosigmoidoscopy is an invasive procedure that provides direct visualization of the rectum, rectosigmoid junction, and lower sigmoid. The indications for this procedure include melena, persistent diarrhea, inflammatory bowel disease, and removal of polyps, tumor, or foreign body.

Premedication: Generally, rectosigmoidoscopy is performed with the infant and young child under sedation (see "Premedication" under "Liver Biopsy"). In the older child, only mild sedation is necessary if he is apprehensive. Preteen and adolescent patients rarely require medication for this procedure. General anesthesia is avoided since the risk of bowel perforation is greater in the patient who is asleep (9).

Diet: No special diet is necessary.

Time: 10 to 15 minutes.

Procedure: The child is placed in a knee chest position. Special proctologic tables are sometimes used that permit the patient to be placed in an inverted position with the head down against a headrest. The left lateral recumbent position may also be satisfactory. Infants may be examined in a supine position with the thighs abducted to the abdomen.

With the child properly positioned and draped, the physician gently spreads the buttocks and performs a digital rectal examination. The patient is then asked to " strain down" while the lubricated instrument is introduced. The obturator is removed and the sigmoidoscope is advanced slowly under direct vision to a depth of 12 cm in infants and 20 to 25 cm in the older child (9). The instrument is gradually withdrawn and the mucosa carefully inspected. Biopsy specimens may be taken or polyps excised. Air insufflation is seldom necessary and increases the patient's discomfort. Cramping sensations may be alleviated somewhat by deep breathing.

Preparation: Patients who have ulcerative colitis or acute diarrhea can be examined without the use of cleansing enemas or laxatives. Such preparation could produce changes in the bowel mucosa that might be misleading. In more routine examinations, children are prepared with a Fleet or saline enema the morning of the examination. The procedure is performed after the child has evacuated the lower bowel. Occasionally, a second enema may be needed if excessive fecal material is encountered during the examination. (9). An explanation of the procedure should be given the child, with a sympathetic understanding of possible embarrassment. Assurance of privacy by careful draping and a matter-of-fact attitude are helpful. The child should be warned that he may feel some cramping, which can be alleviated to some extent by deep breathing or panting "like a puppy." Younger children may benefit from a practice session. The child should be told that he will feel the urge to defecate when the instrument is inserted.

Restraint Necessary: The child will need to maintain the knee chest or lateral recumbent position for the duration of the procedure. Adequate preparation by a reassuring nurse is essential.

Aftercare: The child may resume normal activity and diet after the procedure. The physician should be notified in case of rectal bleeding or abdominal pain. Perforation and bleeding from biopsy sites are rare complications of rectosigmoidoscopy.

SMALL BOWEL BIOPSY

Small bowel biopsy is an invasive procedure used to obtain a sample of intestinal mucosa for examination. The major use of intestinal biopsy is in the differential diagnosis of malabsorption syndromes and other conditions resulting in chronic diarrhea. It is the most important laboratory test for the diagnosis of celiac disease and is of diagnostic value in numerous other conditions including intestinal lymphangiectasis, Whipple's disease, and abetalipoproteinemia.

Premedication: Some physicians prefer to omit sedation; it decreases intestinal motility and thus slows the progress of the biopsy capsule. In most institutions, however, an IM sedative is given 1 hour before the procedure, especially for children between the ages of 2 and 5 years or for irritable infants.

Diet: The child is kept NPO six to eight hours before the procedure, but may have small amounts of water up to 1 hour before.

Consent: An authorization signed by the parent or guardian is necessary.

Time: 45 minutes to 1 hour.

Procedure: A modified Crosby capsule, adapted for pediatric use, or a Carey capsule or most frequently used. The capsule is attached to polyethylene tubing with a 50- to 100-ml tight-fitting syringe.

In small infants the capsule is placed at the base of the tongue and then gently advanced. Cooperative infants will swallow the capsule quickly. The older child may find it easier to swallow the capsule if he is allowed to sit on the edge of a bed or table. Drinking water sometimes helps stimulate swallowing movements. A local anesthetic such as Cetacaine may be given to decrease gagging and to facilitate passage through the pharynx. The tube is then gently advanced to the stomach and the proximal end taped securely to his cheeks. The child is taken to the fluoroscopy room where he is placed on his right side, and the progress of the instrument is monitored under direct vision. When the capsule reaches the first loop of the jejunum, 5 cc of air or saline are flushed through the tubing with a syringe to insure that mucus and debris are flushed out and that the capsule is open. Suction is then applied and maintained for a few seconds, creating a vacuum that sucks mucosa into the capsule. The capsule closes instantly as suction from the syringe is released, cutting the mucosa. Multiple biopsy specimens may be taken before the tube is removed. Once the capsule has been withdrawn, the biopsy specimen should be promptly removed from the capsule. A small piece can be immediately cut off for electron microscope studies, and the remainder placed in formol-saline and examined under the dissecting microscope. Another portion may also be removed before fixation for assay of disaccharidase content (15).

Preparation: Platelet count, prothrombin time, partial thromboplastin time, and bleeding times should be obtained before the biopsy. In generalized malabsorption, the prolonged prothrombin time is treated with intramuscular Vitamin K a few hours before the examination.

The child should be given a simple explanation of the procedure. He should be prepared for the insertion of the biopsy capsule and the attached tube through his mouth and the gagging sensation as it passes down his throat. It usually takes 30 to 40 minutes for peristalsis to carry the capsule through the duodenum. During this time the child lies on his right side and experiences no discomfort. The child should be told that the doctor will be looking at his stomach through the x-ray machine (fluroscopy) several times during the procedure. When the capsule is in the proper position it will remove a tiny piece of the lining of his intestine. This is not painful. Then the tube will be withdrawn and the child may return to his room. If a postbiopsy hematocrit is planned, the child should be prepared for this venipuncture as well. If a sedative was given, the child will be sleepy for several hours.

Restraint Necessary: The child must remain still both when the tube is passed and throughout the procedure. Adequate explanation and sedation are helpful. If these measures are inadequate, a mummy restraint is most effective.

Aftercare: Vital signs should be checked frequently for 2 hours after the procedure. An hematocrit is done 4 to 6 hours later and stools should be checked for blood. If a local pharyngeal anesthetic was used, the child should be placed on his side or abdomen and kept NPO until he is able to swallow safely. A soft diet may be given when normal swallowing control returns.

UPPER GI ENDOSCOPY

Upper GI endoscopy is an invasive procedure that provides direct visualization of the esophagus, stomach, and duodenum.

Fiber endoscopy, an adjunct to roentogenographic examination, is used as a diagnostic tool for gastrointestinal diseases. It can also be used for therapeutic purposes: removal of foreign bodies, esophageal dilatation under visual control, and polypectomy (2,3,4).

The fiberoptic endoscope (Fig. 7-3) permits visualization of previously inaccessible portions of the GI tract. The flexible fiberoptic scope consists of a lens connected by thousands of fiberglass threads to a distal lens at the tip of the endoscope. Images can be transmitted through the fiberglass threads for a distance of one centimeter to several meters in either a straight or a curved line. Cold light from an electric power source is transmitted by another set of fiberglass threads in the scope. The flexible fiberscope has a tip deflection of 180 degrees and is equipped with channels for air insufflation, irrigation of

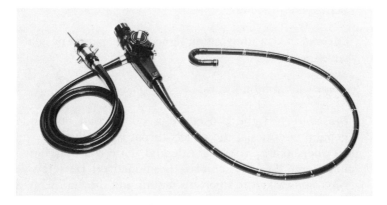

Figure 7-3
Fiberoptic gastroscope. (Photograph courtesy of Olympus Corporation of America, New Hyde Park, New York.)

the lens, suction and passage of instruments for cautery, biopsy, and removal of foreign objects. Photographs can also be taken using the endoscope.

Upper gastrointestinal endoscopy is not performed as frequently in infants and children as in adults. One reason for this is the problem in miniaturization of the equipment. Image quality is obtained in adult scopes by the large number of fibers in the system. The smaller diameter of pediatric scopes results in a smaller image of less quality.

Premedication: Upper GI endoscopy is usually performed under general anesthesia but may be done with sedation alone. General anesthesia is usually preferred for preschoolers and infants. Older children may be sedated with a narcotic with or without atropine IM 30 minutes before the examination. Diazepam (Valium) may also be given by slow IV push immediately before the examination to relax the child and to help him cooperate during the examination. Some physicians also anesthetize the patient's throat with a lidocaine spray or gargle. The exact regime of medication varies between institutions.

Diet: The child should be kept NPO for 6 to 8 hours before the procedure.

Consent: An authorization signed by the parent or guardian is necessary.

Time: 20 to 30 minutes.

Procedure: If the procedure is not carried out under general anesthesia, the child's throat is anesthetized with an anesthetic spray or gargle and diazepam may be administered IV. The child is positioned on his left side. Next he is asked to open his mouth and the endoscope is introduced and advanced slowly, with a mouth guard carefully positioned between the teeth to prevent damage to the instrument. The child is asked to attempt to swallow as the endoscope is passed. The instrument is advanced under direct vision. Inspection of the stomach is optimized by air insufflation. Biopsy specimens may be taken or foreign bodies removed.

Preparation: The child's mouth should be examined for loose teeth that may become dislodged as the endoscope is inserted.

The child should be prepared for the preoperative medication and the drowsy feeling following it. If general anesthesia is planned, a brief description of the endoscopy room and what the child will encounter there before induction of general anesthesia will be helpful. The child should be told he will awaken in the recovery room and then will be returned to his own room. He should also be told that he will be able to eat and play as usual when he is fully awake.

If the child is to be examined without general anesthesia, he should be prepared for the IM premedication or the IV sedative and the drowsy feeling following it. He should also be told that the doctor will "put his throat to sleep" for a short time with a spray medicine or gargle. This medicine may cause his throat and tongue to feel swollen and may make him feel that he is unable to swallow. The child should be told that the lights in the room will be dimmed during the endoscopy procedure. The doctor will place a "bite block" between the child's teeth when he passes the scope to prevent damage to the instrument. The child will feel like gagging while the scope is being passed down his throat. He will be told to "pant like a puppy" and to swallow at this time. When the physician examines the stomach, he may turn the child to different positions and gently press on the abdomen from time to time. At the completion of the examination, the physician will ask the child to hold his breath for a moment while he withdraws the scope. After the procedure, the child may have a sore throat from the endoscope. If diazepam was used, the child may have limited recall of the procedure due to the amnesia that frequently follows administration of this drug. The child will feel sleepy for a few hours until the sedative wears off.

Restraint Necessary: An uncooperative, struggling child would make endoscopy a dangerous procedure, increasing the risk of perforation or bleeding. Adequate sedation and preparation help to increase the child's cooperation. Highly anxious or very young children should be examined under general anesthesia.

Aftercare: The child should be observed closely after the examination, remaining on his side until fully awake to prevent aspiration. Vital signs should be monitored frequently until general anesthesia has worn off.

If sedation and a local anesthetic were used, the child should not be given food or drink for 3 hours after the examination to avoid aspiration. If the child received intravenous diazepam, he may display transitory behavioral disturbances in the recovery period. The child should be allowed to recover from sedation in a quiet, protected environment.

UPPER GI SERIES AND SMALL BOWEL EXAMINATION

The upper GI series and small bowel examination are noninvasive radiologic procedures used to visualize the esophagus, stomach, duodenum, and small intestine.

Premedication: None.

Diet: Most infants should be kept without a feeding 4 or 5 hours before the examination. Older infants and children who are not on a night feeding schedule should be

NPO after going to sleep the evening before the examination.

Time: Upper GI series: 30 minutes
          Small bowel exam: 2 to 4 hours

Procedure: As with any radiologic examination of children, special attention should be directed to the problem of radiation protection. Whenever possible, the gonadal area should be protected by lead shielding.

The major problem encountered in the upper GI examination of young children is the reluctance of the patient to drink the contrast media. Young infants, hungry from fasting, will readily take barium from a nursing bottle if the nipple opening has been slightly enlarged. Some radiologists prefer to pass a nasogastric tube into the infant's stomach and inject barium directly.

The older infant and young child, usually between the ages of 1 to 3 years, are the most challenging to examine because of their reluctance to drink the barium. Having the child sit on the examiner's lap as he forcefully feeds the child through a cup is usually the most successful technique.

The older child is usually cooperative, especially if the barium is flavored. Children in this age group are usually able to follow the radiologist's instructions during the procedure.

As the barium is ingested, the radiologist observes the filling of the stomach under fluoroscopy, turning the child to right and left oblique positions. Following this, the tumbler of barium is taken from the child and the radiologist observes the progression of the barium and applies intermittent compression to the abdomen with his gloved hand. X-ray films are usually first taken with the table in a vertical position with the child standing, followed by films in the supine and prone positions.

In the small bowel examination, the child drinks another cup of barium and sequential films are made at half-hour intervals, unless the initial fluoroscopy revealed an unusually rapid transit time. Each film is developed and inspected immediately to determine the progress of the barium and to determine if additional fluoroscopy and spot films are necessary.

Preparation: No physical preparation other than dietary restriction is necessary. The child should be told that while in the x-ray room he will be asked to drink a cup of barium, a chocolate- or strawberry-flavored liquid the consistency of a malted milk. Then the doctor will take pictures of his stomach. If a small bowel examination is also planned, the child should be prepared for the period of time he must wait between films. The child should also be prepared for the position changes of the tilting table and be assured that he will not fall.

Restraint Necessary: The child must remain still while the spot films are being taken. Adequate explanation will enable most older children to do this without restraint. The child should be adequately secured to the tilting x-ray table since it moves from a vertical to a horizontal position. The use of a mummy board is impractical for immobilization of the infant because of the need to turn him from a supine to a prone position. Instead, personnel or parents protected with lead aprons may hold the child still while the films are taken.

Aftercare: Castor oil or milk of magnesia should be given to eliminate the barium. The child should be followed closely to make sure that the barium is expelled. Constipation and impaction may occur if barium is allowed to remain in the colon. The child's stool will be white for 24 to 48 hours after the examination. Parents and older children should be informed of changes in stool appearance to prevent undue worry. The child may eat a regular diet after the x-ray films are taken. Liberal fluid intake is encouraged to promote the passage of barium.

REFERENCES

1. Margulis AR, Burhenne HJ *Alimentary Tract Roentgenology.* St Louis, CV Mosby Co, 1973.
2. Cadranel S, Rodesch P, Peeters, et al: Fiberendoscopy of the Gastrointestinal Tract in Children. *Am. J Dis Child* 131:41, 1977.
3. Gans S, Ament M, Christie D, et al: Pediatric Endoscopy with Flexible Fiberscopes. *J Pediatr Surg* 10:375, 1975.
4. Daum F, Zucker P, Boley et al: Colonoscopic Polypectomy in Children. *Am. J Dis Child* 131:566, 1977.
5. Hansen LK: Coloscopy, An Analysis of 120 Cases with Special Regards to Technique. *Endoscopy* 5:77, 1973.
6. Rossini FP: *Atlas of Coloscopy.* New York, Piccin Medical Books, 1975.
7. Smith JH, Roberts G, Ohan A: Fiberoptic Colonscopy. *Tex Med* 72:90, 1976.
8. Marks G, Moses ML: The Clinical Application of Flexible Fiberoptic Colonoscopy. *Surg Clin North Am* 53:737, 1973.
9. Roy CC, Silverman A: *Pediatric Clinical Gastroenterology.* St Louis CV Mosby Co, 1975.
10. Skydell B, Crowder AS: *Diagnostic Procedures.* Boston, Little, Brown & Company, 1975, p. 93.
11. Skydell B, Crowder AS: *Diagnostic Procedures.* Boston, Little, Brown & Company, 1975, p. 93.
12. Lavelle MI, Owen JP, McNulty S et al: Initial Experience of Percutaneous Transhepatic Cholangiography Using a Fine Gauge Needle. *Clin Radio,* 28:453, 1977.
13. Okuda K, Tanikawa K. Emura T et al: Nonsurgical Percutaneous Transhepatic Cholangiography Diagnostic Significance in Medical Problems of the Liver. *Digestive Diseases* 19:21, 1977.
14. Zinberg S, Berk JE, Plasencia H: Percutaneous Transhepatic Cholangiography: Its Use and Limitations. *Am. J Digestive Dis* 10:154, 1969.
15. Walker-Smith J: *Diseases of the Small Intestine in Childhood.* New York, John Wiley & Sons, Inc. 1975.

BIBLIOGRAPHY

Allegra G, et al: *Gastroscopy with the Fiberscope.* New York, Piccin Medical Books, 1971.
Ament ME, Christie DL: Upper Gastrointestinal Fiberoptic En-

doscopy in Pediatric Patients. *Gastroenterology* 72:1244, 1977.

Beck, RN, Clemett AR: *Radiology of the Gallbladder and Bile Ducts.* Philadelphia, WB Saunders Co, 1977.

Belinsky I, Shinga H, Wolff W: Colonfiberoscopy: Technique in Colon Examination. *Am J Nurs* 73:306, 1973.

Bohlman T, Katon R, Lipshutz G, et al: Fiberoptic Pansigmoidoscopy. *Gastroenterology* 72:644, 1977.

Cadranel S, Rodesch P, Peeters JP et al: Fiberendoscopy of the Gastrointestional Tract in Children. *Am J Dis Child* 131:41, 1977.

Daum F, Zucker P, Boley SJ et al: Colonoscopic Polysectomy in Children. *Am J Dis Child* 131:566, 1977.

Demling L, Otterjam R, Elsten K: *Endoscopy and Biopsy of the Esophagus and Stomach.* Philadelphia, WB Saunders Co, 1972.

Gans S, Berci G: Advances in Endoscopy of Infants and Children. *J Pediatr Surg* 6:199, 1971.

Gans S, Ament N, Christie DL, et al: Pediatric Endoscopy with Flexible Fiberscopes. *J Pediatr Surg* 10:375, 1975.

Hansen LK: Coloscopy, An Analysis of 120 Cases with Special Regards to Technique. *Endoscopy* 5:77, 1973.

Hines C, Ferrante W, Davis W: Percutaneous Transhepatic Cholangiography, *Digestive Diseases* 17:868, 1972.

Lavelle MI, Owen JP, McNulty S, et al: Initial Experience of Percutaneous Transhepatic Cholangiography Using a Fine Gauge Needle. *Clin Radiol* 28:453, 1977.

Margulis AR, Burhenne HJ: *Alimentary Tract Roentgenology.* St Louis, CV Mosby Co, 1973.

Marks G, Moses ML: The Clinical Application of Flexible Fiberoptic Colonoscopy. *Surg Clin North Am* 53:737, 1973.

Okuda K, Tanikawa K, Emura T et al: Nonsurgical Percutaneous Transhepatic Cholangiography—Diagnostic Significant in Medical Problems of the Liver. *Digestive Diseases* 19:21, 1974.

Rossini FP *Atlas of Coloscopy.* New York, Piccin Medical Books, 1975.

Roy CC, Silverman A: *Pediatric Clinical Gastroenterology.* St Louis, CV Mosby Co, 1975.

Schapiro R *Clinical Radiology of the Pediatric Abdomen and Gastro intentinal Tract.* Baltimore, Md, University Park Press, 1976.

Schiller KF, Salmon PR: *Modern Topics in Gastrointestional Endoscopy.* Chicago, Year Book Medical Publishers, 1976.

Singleton EB, Wagner M, Dultor R, et al: Radiology of the Alimentary Tract in Infants and Children, ed 2. Philadelphia, WB Saunders Co, 1977.

Skydell G, Crowder AS: *Diagnostic Procedures.* Boston, Little, Brown & Co., 1975.

Smith JH, Roberts G, Ohan A, et al: Fiberoptic Colonoscopy. *Tex Med* 72:90, 1976.

Tilkian SM: *Clinical Implications of Laboratory Tests.* St Louis, CV Mosby Co, 1975.

Urakami H, Saki H, Kishi S: Endoscopie Retrograde Cholangiopan creatography (ERCP) Performed in Children. *Endoscopy* 9:8b, 1977.

Walker-Smith J: *Diseases of the Small intestine in Childhood.* New York, John Wiley & Sons, 1975.

Wayne JD: Endoscopic Retrograde Cholangiopancreatography in Infants. *Am J Gastroenterology* May 1976, p 461.

Zinberg S, Berk JE, Plasencia H: Percutaneous Transhepatic Cholangiography: Its Use and Limitations. *Am J Digestive Diseases* 10:154, 1965.

8

Urologic Diagnostic Procedures

CYSTOURETHROSCOPY

Cystoscopy (cystourethroscopy) is an invasive procedure used to directly visualize the bladder, urethra, and urethral orifices. Cystoscopy is useful for investigating congenital abnormalities or acquired lesions in the bladder and lower urinary tract, or for performing ureteral catheterization.

Premedication: An IM preoperative sedative will be administered to enhance the general anesthesia.

Diet: The child may be given clear liquids until 6 to 8 hours before the procedure and then is kept NPO.

Consent: An authorization signed by the parent or guardian is necessary.

Time: 15 to 45 minutes depending on the patient's pathology and the degree of difficulty encountered inserting the cystoscope.

Procedure: An intravenous infusion is started and anesthesia induced. The patient is placed on the cystoscopy table in the lithotomy position. The area around the urethral orifice is cleansed with an antiseptic solution and sterile drapes are applied. The lubricated cystoscope is inserted into the bladder through the urethra. Sterile fluid is instilled into the bladder to promote visualization. The bladder, urethra, and ureteral orifices are inspected. Biopsy of tissue or removal of calculi or foreign bodies may be performed at this time. Ureteral catheterization and retrograde pyelography may also be done in conjunction with this procedure. When the examination is completed, the cystoscope is removed.

Preparation: The child should be prepared for the period of time he will be NPO, the preoperative injection, and the sleepy feeling following it. He should be told about the trip to the operating room, the sight of the cystoscopy room with strange equipment, sounds, smells, and people attired in masks and gowns. He will feel pain during venipuncture, and the drowsy feeling following the "stick." The child should be reassured that if he goes to sleep he will wake up after the procedure. Also, since many young children fear discomfort during and after urologic procedures, this must be discussed. The child should be told he will be asleep during the procedure and that the doctor will look at his bladder during this time. After the procedure the child will awaken in the "wake-up" room and will be taken to his own room as soon as he is fully awake.

Aftercare: Vital signs should be checked when the child returns to his room and every 30 minutes to 1 hour until stable. Careful monitoring of urinary output is essential to detect urinary retention caused by edema. Any hematuria should also be noted. Fluids should be encouraged. Cool perineal compresses or warm tub baths may be soothing.

INTRAVENOUS PYELOGRAM

The intravenous pyelogram (IVP) is a radiologic procedure used to provide information about the kidneys, ureters, and bladder. A contrast medium is injected intravenously and is excreted by the kidneys, making the urinary tract visible on x-ray films. Size, shape, and position of the organs are revealed by an IVP, in addition to the rate of excretion of radiopaque media.

Premedication: None.

Diet: The child is given a light dinner the evening before the test and then is offered only clear liquids until midnight. The child should remain NPO from midnight until the examination. The slight dehydration afforded by this restriction facilitates concentration of the contrast media and is necessary for good visualization. Such fluid restriction may be dangerous, however, for a sick child younger than 2 years of age. Some radiology departments recommend no preparation be used for intravenous pyelography in infants, other than withholding solid food and allowing only one bottle on the morning of the examination.

Consent: An authorization signed by the parent or guardian is necessary.

Procedure: The child is placed in a supine position and a preliminary scout film is taken. A small amount of radiopaque material is injected into an antecubital vein. If no hypersensitivity is evident within a minute or so, the remainder is injected. A carbonated beverage may be given after the contrast material is injected. Gas in the stomach provides a "window" that promotes visualization of the kidneys. Films are usually taken 5, 10, and 15 minutes after the injection. The last film may be taken with the child in an upright position after he has voided. This provides additional information about renal mobility and the ability of the kidneys and ureters to empty. The number of films taken, the interval between films, and the positioning of the patient may vary. Fluoroscopy may also be used. In a modification of the test, the timed sequence IVP, films are made every minute for 5 minutes after the injection. Another modification, the drip infusion IVP, requires the contrast material to be mixed with an equal volume of IV solution (2 ml per pound of body weight, up to 300 ml). The solution is infused over a period of 5 to 10 minutes. This affords a denser opacification and may be used for the patient who has mild azotemia with a BUN of 40 to 50.

Untoward reactions to the contrast media have ranged from minor (nausea, emesis, flushing, and urticaria) to severe (bronchospasm, chest pain, edema of the glottis, and cardiac arrhythmias). Although severe reactions are rare, emergency drugs should be readily available, including epinephrine, an antihistamine, a sedative, a steroid preparation, and oxygen.

Because of the radiation hazard, the gonads of males should be protected by a lead covering. In females, the lower half of the abdomen should be covered after visualization of the lower urinary tract.

Preparation: A Fleets enema and a mild cathartic are administered the evening before the test to clear the bowel of feces and gas that would obscure the renal outline. The enema should be explained fully to the child, because this procedure may be seen as threatening as the IVP itself. The child should void immediately before the procedure since urine will dilute the contrast material and make visualization of the bladder difficult.

The child should also be prepared for the trip to the x-ray department, the sight of the x-ray machine and table, positioning in a supine position on the x-ray table, a preliminary abdominal x-ray picture, pain during venipuncture, a stinging or burning sensation as the radiopaque material is injected, and the necessity of holding very still while the pictures are being taken. The child may move around on the table and use slightly more mobile methods of coping with his anxiety between films. The child should be told that several pictures will be taken and he must wait on the x-ray table between pictures. The intervals between pictures may seem interminable to the child. Support must be provided during this waiting period. Reassure the child that he will not be left alone. The contrast material often produces side effects such as a generalized feeling of warmth or nausea. The child should be reassured that these sensations will last only a short time.

Aftercare: No physical aftercare.

Restraint Necessary: Restraint will probably be needed most during venipuncture. The child must remain still while the films are being taken. Usually if a child older than 3 years has been properly prepared, he will be able to do this without restraint. If restraint is necessary, however, it will be only for a few seconds while the films are being taken. Someone should remain near the child throughout the procedure. Lead garments will protect personnel from radiation.

Interpretation: Renal size is revealed by the IVP. Bilaterally enlarged renal shadows are seen in nephrotic syndrome, acute pyelonephritis, polycystic disease, and leukemic infiltration of the kidneys. Abnormally small kidneys may suggest chronic glomerulonephritis, chronic pyelonephritis, or congenital dysplasia. There should be no more than 1.5 cm difference in size between the two kidneys. A single enlarged kidney may be the result of partial ureteral obstruction, inflammatory disease, bleeding, tumor, or unilateral cystic disease. A unilaterally small kidney suggests dysplasia, ischemic atrophy, or unilateral chronic pyelonephitis. (1).

LABORATORY TESTS

Examination of the Urine: Urinalysis is the least expensive and most widely useful test for the evaluation of renal disease. A routine urinalysis includes determination of pH, specific gravity, protein, glucose, ketones, and a microscopic examination for cells, casts, crystals, and bacteria.

To insure accuracy, the specimen must be carefully obtained and analyzed as soon as possible. A freshly voided morning specimen is ideal for urinalysis, since this urine is generally concentrated and acidic. During the daytime hours a randomly collected specimen is satisfactory, but forcing a child to drink large quantities of water in order to obtain a urine specimen should be avoided. The urine obtained in such a manner would be dilute and significant results may be obscured.

Urine Culture: A urine culture may be obtained by a "clean catch," catheterization, or suprapubic aspiration. In the "clean catch" method, scrupulous cleansing of the area is imperative. Special attention must be given to cleansing the perineum, spreading the labia in females, and obtaining the specimen midstream. Accuracy of the culture depends on meticulous technique. If a sterile pediatric urine collection bag is used, it should be checked frequently for spills and contamination. If the infant has not voided after 45 minutes, cleansing should be repeated and the bag reapplied.

Catheterization may be used if the child is unable to void or if two or more clean catch specimens have yielded positive results. Aseptic technique is essential to prevent contamination of the specimen or introduction of microorganisms into the bladder.

Suprapubic aspiration precludes the problem of urethral contamination and is a relatively safe procedure in experienced hands. It is particularly useful in infants because of the difficulty in obtaining clean catch specimens and the trauma involved in catheterization (1). To insure a successful aspiration, the bladder should be full enough to be palpated above the symphysis. The urethra is compressed manually (through the rectum in females) and the suprapubic area is cleansed with an antiseptic solution. A 1½ to 2 inch, 21 gauge needle is inserted approximately 1 cm above the symphysis. The bladder is usually entered at a depth of about 1 inch, and urine can be gently aspirated at this point. Transient hematuria is the most frequent complication. Bowel perforation with resulting peritonitis, abscess formation in the needle tract, and bleeding have been reported infrequently (1). The chances of serious complications are increased if the bladder is not adequately full or if the bowel is distended with gas.

Any urine specimen for culture should be sent to the laboratory immediately or refrigerated. Urine may be kept in the refrigerator at 8° for up to 48 hours without significant bacterial growth (2).

Addis Count: The Addis count provides an estimation of the rate of excretion of red cells, white cells, and casts in the urine. Fluids are withheld for a period of time to insure concentration of urine. A 12-hour urine specimen is then collected. Normal values per 12 hours for the Addis count are listed in the Appendix. Although refrigerated urine is satisfactory for bacterial analysis, casts and other formed elements begin to deteriorate after about 3 hours; thus fresh urine is essential for accurate results.

Serum BUN and Creatinine: Urea and creatinine are nitrogenous wastes that are normally removed by the kidney. The serum values of these products do not become elevated significantly until the renal filtration rate is reduced by about 60%. To detect less severe renal impairment, clearance measurements are used. The BUN level varies according to protein and fluid intake and, therefore, is generally less accurate than the creatinine measurement, which is little affected by diet (1).

Urea and Creatinine Clearance: The efficiency of glomerular filtration may be determined with reasonable accuracy by a urea and/or creatinine clearance test. These substances are present in the plasma in relatively stable concentrations and may be measured in timed urine specimens. Their clinical value lies in the fact that they are freely filtered at the glomerulus and are only slightly secreted and reabsorbed by the tubules. Therefore, the quantity of creatinine appearing in the urine during a given period will equal the quantity filtered during the same period, and if the plasma concentration is also measured, the filtration rate can be determined (1).

Loss of urine (spills, patient or practitioner error) is the most common cause of inaccurate results of the clearance test. For this reason temporary catheterization is indicated for children who are not bladder trained, especially when creatinine clearance measurement is critical. A blood sample is taken at the midpoint of urine collection. Normal creatinine clearance is 110 ml/min/1.73 sq m. Normal urea clearance is 70 ml/min/1.73 sq m.

RENAL BIOPSY

Renal biopsy is an invasive procedure used to obtain histologic and microscopic information about the glomeruli and tubules. The information obtained from this procedure is valuable in guiding the treatment of steroid-resistant nephrotic syndrome, systemic lupus erythematosus, chronic glomerulonephritis, unexplained hypertension, and other renal diseases where histologic information is needed.

Premedication: The child is premedicated with an IM sedative 45 minutes before the procedure.

Diet: The child is kept NPO 4 to 6 hours before this procedure.

Consent: An authorization signed by the parent or guardian is necessary.

Time: 20 minutes.

Procedure: The child is placed on the x-ray table in a prone position with a radiolucent cushion under his abdomen. A contrast medium is injected intravenously, and the kidney is located by fluoroscopy using an image intensifier. Usually, the right kidney is selected in order to avoid puncture of the spleen and major vessels located on the left side. The area is cleansed with an antiseptic solution and draped with sterile towels. A local anesthetic is infiltrated subcutaneously. A small skin incision is made and the biopsy needle with stilette in place is then introduced. Correct placement of the biopsy needle is checked radiologically. The kidney is pushed downward by contraction of the diaphragm, during each respiration, and this movement is used to confirm the correct placement of the biopsy needle. If the needle is in the kidney, its tip will move synchronously with the renal shadow during respirations. When proper placement has been accomplished, the stilette is removed and the prongs inserted into the outer needle. A specimen about the size of a pencil lead is taken quickly and the needle removed. The specimen is divided into a part for histologic study and another part for electron microscopy and immunofluorescent staining. After the biopsy needle is removed, firm pressure must be held over the site for 10 minutes to prevent bleeding.

Preparation: Before the procedure a careful check should be made of the child's hemaglobin concentration (which should be seven grams or more) and of the blood clotting mechanism (platelet count, bleeding time, coagulation time, prothrombin time, partial thromboplastin time, and thromboplastin generation test; see Appendix B for normal values). The child's blood pressure should be controlled before biopsy, as severe hypertension increases the risk of hemorrhage. Blood should be typed, crossmatched, and held on call beforehand. This procedure is contraindicated in the presence of a solitary kidney or a bleeding tendency.

The child should be prepared for premedication and a drowsy feeling following it. The child will be taken to the x-ray department where he will experience pain during venipuncture, a cold feeling when the skin is cleansed with an antiseptic solution, a stinging or burning sensation when local anesthetic is injected into the subcutaneous tissues, a feeling of pressure when the biopsy needle is advanced, withdrawal of the needle as soon as the biopsy material has been aspirated, and firm pressure at the puncture site for 5 to 10 minutes. The child must understand the necessity of remaining absolutely still during the procedure. Following the biopsy, the child will be returned to his room where he will stay in bed for 24 hours. After the procedure the child will be encouraged to drink a large amount of fluid and to save all voided urine. He may experience some flank pain for a day or so.

Restraint Necessary: It is imperative that the child remain absolutely still during the biopsy. Premedication and proper preparation will aid in accomplishing this. Because of the danger of kidney laceration and subsequent hemorrhage in the uncooperative child, this procedure is usually limited to older children. Younger or especially apprehensive children unable to remain still during the procedure may require general anesthesia.

Aftercare: Bleeding is the major complication. The child should remain in bed 24 hours after biopsy. Pulse and blood pressure should be checked frequently (every 15 minutes for 2 hours, every half-hour for 2 hours; every hour for 4 hours, and then every 3 hours). A high fluid intake should be encouraged. Urine should be observed for hematuria. Microscopic hematuria is common, but grossly bloody urine should be reported.

URODYNAMICS

Urodynamics is the term used for a group of invasive tests that yield graphic recordings of intrabladder pressure, urinary flow rate, and anal muscle or sphincter activity. Such data may be valuable for diagnosis and treatment of children exhibiting recurrent urinary tract infections, daytime wetting, encopresis, or abnormal renal x-ray films with evidence of hydronephrosis or residual urine.

MICTURATION STUDY

Premedication: The child is premedicated with a routine preoperative medication before the micturation prep (cystoscopy), which is performed the day before the micturation study. No medication is given before the micturation study itself.

Diet: Same as for cystoscopy before the micturation prep. No restrictions after cystoscopy.

Consent: An authorization signed by the parent or guardian is necessary.

Time: 30 minutes for the micturation prep (cystoscopy). 15 minutes to 1 hour for the micturation study, depending on the data needed.

Procedure: The child undergoes a cystoscopic examination under general anesthesia the day before testing. After examining the bladder, the physician inserts a suprapubic catheter. Four stainless wire electrodes are inserted through the skin close to the anus into the anal and urethral sphincter muscles. These wires are then taped to the inside of the child's thighs to prevent the wires from being accidentally withdrawn. Since this does not secure the wires completely, the patient must remain on bedrest until the micturation study. (The patient will be transported to the urodynamics laboratory by stretcher the next day.)

The micturation study is performed the day after the cystoscopy to allow the child to recover from medications given before the cystoscopy and to adjust to the possible discomfort of the wires. The child should be encouraged to eat meals as usual that day.

During the micturation study the child sits on a special toilet that measures urinary flow rate (Fig. 8-1). The four

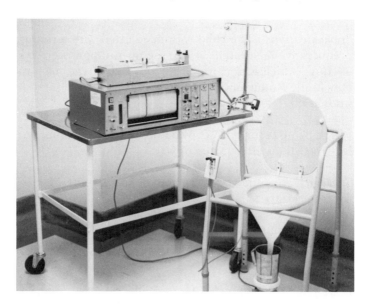

Figure 8-1
Equipment used in urodynamic studies. The machine graphically records intrabladder pressure, urinary flow rate, and muscle activity. The syringe above the graphic recorder instills sterile water into the bladder at a precise rate of flow.

wire electrodes are connected to a ground plate on the inner thigh near the groin area to measure muscle activity. The suprapubic catheter, connected to sterile water from an IV setup, is attached to a pressure transducer to measure bladder pressure.

Sterile water is then instilled into the bladder at a set rate of flow until the patient states he has a strong urge to urinate. The flow of sterile water is then turned off and the patient voids. During voiding flow rate, bladder pressure, and muscle activity are graphically recorded. If a rectal catheter has been inserted, it also records abdominal pressure. After the child has voided, the procedure is repeated two or three times in order to obtain the normal bladder pressure.

When the results have been obtained, the child is returned to the stretcher. The suprapubic catheter is removed and a sterile 3×3 inch gauze placed over the tiny pubic incision and held securely with micropore tape. The anal wire electrodes are gently removed. The child is returned to his room by stretcher.

Other urodynamic tests frequently performed are urethral pressure profile, cystometrogram, and flow rate.

Urethral Pressure Profile: This is a graphic recording of urethral pressure. A small, straight, sterile catheter is inserted into the urethra using sterile technique. It is slowly withdrawn and the pressures inside the urethra are measured from the bladder neck to the meatus.

Cystometrogram: This is a graphic recording of intrabladder pressure. With the child lying on a stretcher, an indwelling catheter is introduced into the bladder using sterile technique. Carbon dioxide is instilled into the bladder through the catheter and the bladder pressure is recorded. If a recording of anal muscle activity is desired, a small anal plug electrode is inserted into the rectum.

Flow Rate: This is a graphic recording of a timed voiding

flow rate. This simple test is usually performed on an outpatient basis. The child is instructed to void into a special toilet that measures flow rate. It is important for the child to be well hydrated before the test.

Preparation: The child should be prepared for the micturation prep as he would be for a cystoscopy (see "Cystourethroscopy"). He should also be told that when he awakes in the recovery room, he will have one small tube in his lower abdomen (suprapubic catheter) and four small wires in his rectum that will be taped to his inner thigh. It should be stressed to him that it is very important for these wires and tube to stay in place until the test the next day, so he must stay in bed until then. He may sit up in bed and turn from side to side, but he cannot get out of bed. No rectal temperatures are to be taken. The child should be encouraged to eat meals as usual that day.

The next day the child will be taken to the lab on a stretcher. He will sit on a special toilet (Fig. 8-1). The four wire electrodes will be connected to a machine, and the suprapubic catheter will be connected to a special bottle of water. Water will run from the bottle into his bladder and make him feel that he must urinate. The fluid is then turned off, and he may void in the special toilet. He must remember that he cannot have a bowel movement in this toilet. After he has voided, the procedure may be repeated several times. The child should be prepared for the fact that several people will be watching as he voids. Psychologic inhibitions may be a problem, especially with older children. When the test is completed the child will be returned to the stretcher for removal of the catheter and wires. There will be a brief stinging sensation as they are removed. Removal of the tape on the thighs may also be uncomfortable. A small bandage will be placed on his abdomen. The child will then be returned to his room.

Aftercare: The small abdominal dressing should be kept clean and dry until it is removed the next day. The child may be sent home immediately after the micturation study.

VOIDING CYSTOURETHROGRAPHY

Voiding cystourethrography is an invasive radiologic procedure used to visualize the lower urinary tract during micturation. This procedure is indicated for children with recurrent urinary tract infections, neurogenic bladder, or lower urinary tract obstruction.

Premedication: None.

Diet: No restriction necessary.

Consent: An authorization signed by the parent or guardian is necessary.

Time: 30 minutes.

Procedure: Before the procedure the child is encouraged to empty his bladder. The child is then catheterized and the bladder emptied completely. Any residual urine is measured and a culture is obtained. Radiopaque material is then slowly introduced through the catheter. The amount of material used varies from 75 ml in infants to 200 ml in older children. The catheter is removed after the introduction of the contrast material. Infants usually begin voiding as soon as the bladder fills enough to produce discomfort. In older children, filling is usually stopped when the child begins to complain of fullness. Films are taken during and after voiding, usually using fluoroscopy. The first film is taken with the child in a supine position to provide an anteroposterior view. Films are also taken with the child in the left and right semilateral of the oblique positions. The final exposure, made after the child has completely emptied his bladder, is to show if any residual medium has remained in the bladder or has refluxed into the renal pelvis. Cinefluoroscopy is sometimes used but entails more radiation exposure than conventional fluoroscopy with spot films.

Preparation: A simple explanation of the procedure and its purpose should be given to the child and parents. The child should be prepared for the discomfort of catheterization, since this is the most threatening part of the procedure. The child will experience a feeling of fullness and an urge to void as the contrast material is being introduced through the catheter. The necessity of remaining still during catheterization and while the x-ray films are being taken should be explained. The child should be told that there will be people present to help him hold still.

Restraint Necessary: Accurate filming and visualization are possible only if the child remains still. In young children, immobilzation during this procedure may be best accomplished by using the "mummy restraint." (see Appendix A).

Aftercare: Watch for fever and chills, signs of bacteremia which may be precipitated by instrumentation in infected children. Liberal oral fluids and cool perineal compresses will promote comfort.

Interpretation: Among the most significant pathologic entities detected by this procedure are vesicoureteral reflux and posterior urethral valvular obstruction in males. Abnormalities of the anatomy of the urethra and bladder such as abnormal size or contour, bladder diverticula or fistulae may also be detected. Incomplete evacuation and filling defects may be noted.

REFERENCES

1. James JA: *Renal Disease in Childhood,* ed 3. St. Louis, CV Mosby Co, 1976.
2. Lilly A: *The Tailored Urogram.* Chicago, Year Book Medical Publishers, Inc, 1973.

BIBLIOGRAPHY

Bauer KM: *Cystoscopic Diagnosis.* Philadelphia, Lea & Febiger, 1969.

James JA: *Renal Disease in Childhood,* ed 3. St Louis, CV Mosby Co, 1976.

Kory M, Waife SO: *Kidney and Urinary Tract Infections.* Indianapolis, Lilly Research Laboratories, 1972.

Lilli A: *The Tailored Urogram.* Chicago, Year Book Medical Publishers, Inc, 1973.

Scott BF: "Uroflowmetry." *Urology Times* 4(1): 1, 1976.

Scott, BF: "Micturation Patterns." *Urology Times* 4(1):5, 1976.

Scott BF: "Cystometry: The Reflex Hammer of the Urologist." *Urology Times* 4(1):7, 1976.

Scott BF: "Urethral Pressure Profile." *Urology Times* 4(5):10 1976.

Williams DI: *Urology in Childhood.* New York, Springer-Verlag, New York, Inc, 1971.

Witten DM, Myers G, Utz D: *Clinical Urography,* Vol 1, ed 4. WB Saunders Co, 1977.

9

Ophthalmologic Diagnostic Procedures

CORNEAL STAINING

Corneal staining is a noninvasive technique useful in evaluating the integrity of the corneal epithelium. Such evaluation is valuable in the diagnosis of foreign bodies, abrasions, and inflammations of the cornea.

Time: 5 minutes.

Procedure: The child is seated comfortably and asked to look at an object directly in front of him. Anesthetic eye drops may be instilled. A fluorescein paper strip is moistened with sterile saline and touched to the conjunctiva. A thin film of fluorescein dye spreads over the corneal surface, revealing abnormal tissue or breaks in integrity that are stained by the dye. A blue light is used to detect "bright spots" or breaks in the corneal epithelium.

Preparation: No physical preparation needed.

Aftercare: No physical aftercare is needed, unless anesthetic eye drops were instilled. The local anesthetic wears off in approximately 30 minutes, during which time the child's hands and other objects must be kept away from the eyes to avoid injury.

ELECTRORETINOGRAPHY

Electroretinography (ERG) is a noninvasive procedure useful in the evaluation of retinal function. When a flash of light falls on the retina, rapid changes occur in the resting potential of the retina. Recordings of these electric potentials provide evidence of retinal integrity. Electroretinography gives no information about the optic nerve but can determine if optic atrophy is retinal in origin. It is useful in the diagnosis of some retinal diseases, providing an objective method of investigating the outer retinal layers where ophthalmoscopic examination is impossible.

Premedication: Children younger than 7 years old may require general anesthesia, in which case a routine preoperative sedative would be given 30 to 45 minutes before the procedure.

Mydriatic cycloplegic eye drops are instilled before examination to dilate the pupils. Cyclogyl drops are administered 30 to 40 minutes before the procedure, one drop in each eye, 5 minutes apart. The drops may sting briefly and cause an unusual taste in the mouth. These sensations last only a few minutes. When atropine ointment is the cycloplegic of choice, it is administered at home three times a day for two days before the examination.

Diet: If general anesthesia is to be used, the child should be kept NPO 4 to 6 hours before the procedure to prevent vomiting and possible aspiration of gastric contents.

Consent: An authorization signed by the parent or guardian is necessary if general anesthesia is used.

Time: 45 minutes to 1 hour.

Procedure: The child is placed in a comfortable supine position. If contact lens electrodes are used, topical anesthetic eye drops and methylcellulose eye drops are instilled before inserting the two contact lenses. Two small skin electrodes taped near the orbital rim may be substituted for the lens electrodes. A neutral electrode is taped to the skin above the bridge of the nose after cleansing the skin and applying electrolyte jelly. The child is instructed to keep both eyes open, to look steadily at an overhead point, and not to blink during the test. For accurate results, the eyes must be adapted to light and darkness. Light adaptation may be achieved by asking the child to look at a brightly lit screen for 5 minutes. Light-adapted responses are then elicited with stroboscopic flashes at controlled intensity and speed. When satisfactory light-adapted tracings have been recorded, the room light is extinguished and dark-adapted responses to flashes of light are recorded at 1, 3, 5, 9, 15, and 25 minutes, or other determined intervals. The child may close his eyes during the longer intervals between flashes. The exact sequence of test conditions varies among institutions. Preferably a parent remains in the testing room with the child.

The electric potentials picked up by the electrodes are amplified and then recorded on an inkwriter, displayed on and photographed from an oscilloscope, or recorded by a computer or tape.

Visual evoked potential (VEP) may be obtained in conjunction with the ERG. Visual evoked potential is a measure of the amount of electric activity produced at the occipital cortex by light stimulation of the eyes. It tests the continuity of the visual pathway between the eye and the brain and is used to determine the exact location of lesions of the visual pathway. The VEP is usually recorded with the child sitting to prevent movement of the electrodes and resultant artifacts. Scalp electrodes are placed over the occiput and the child is instructed to look steadily at a screen on which a repetitive flashing stimulus is shown. Rigid fixation on the screen is not essential. Electric impulses are recorded and fed into a computer.

Preparation: The child's face should be washed to remove skin oils in the areas to be used for electrode contact. A simple explanation of the procedure and its purpose should be given to the child and parents. If contact lens electrodes are used, anesthetic eye drops will be instilled immediately before the procedure. This is omitted if small skin electrodes are substituted for contact lens electrodes. A neutral electrode will be taped to the forehead and the contact lens electrodes will be inserted into both eyes. The child will be asked to keep both eyes open and not to blink during the test. Bright lights of different colors will flash for a short period of time and then all the lights in the room will be turned off for approximately 30 minutes. Bright lights will flash occasionally during this time period. A parent may stay in the test room with the child during the test.

Aftercare: The child's cornea should be protected from trauma for 30 to 45 minutes until the effects of the local anesthetic wear off. The child's hands and other objects should be kept away from the eyes. Elbow restraints may be necessary for infants. Pupil dilation may cause the eyes to be extremely sensitive to bright light for a few hours. Wearing dark glasses may increase comfort. The electrode jelly should be washed from the child's hair after the procedure.

EYE ULTRASONOGRAPHY

Ultrasonography of the eye can provide useful clinical information in the presence of corneal opacities, cataracts, or vitreous hemorrhage, conditions that usually obscure visualization by other methods.

Premedication: If the procedure is to be performed under general anesthesia, a preoperative sedative will be given 30 to 45 minutes before the procedure.

Diet: If the procedure is to be performed under general anesthesia, the child should be kept NPO overnight or 4 to 6 hours before the procedure to prevent vomiting and possible aspiration of gastric contents.

Time: 10 to 30 minutes, depending on the purpose of the study.

Procedure: Two types of diagnostic ultrasound are used in ophthalmology: A-mode and B-mode. In the A-mode unit the transducer is placed directly on the cornea or sclera with the use of a coupling medium such as methylcellulose to provide an airtight seal. In uncooperative children the transducer may be placed on the closed lid rather than on the cornea, but this decreases the accuracy of measuring ocular dimension (1). Local anesthetic eye drops are instilled first, then methylcellulose. The transducer is placed on the eye or eyelid and moved in different directions across the eye. The echoes are displayed by A-mode on the oscilloscope screen, and significant information is photographed.

B-mode scanning is very precise. With hand-held B-scanners, the transducer is most often placed on the closed eyelid. Occasionally, however, water immersion of the eye and orbit may be performed. General anesthesia may be necessary for infants and uncooperative children if water immersion is used. The child is placed supine on the examination table and a waterproof drape is secured around the orbit with collodion. The eye is left exposed. Anesthetic eye drops are instilled and the child is asked to look up and down and not to blink. An eyelid retractor is applied. This is not uncomfortable because of the anesthetic eye drops. The eye is covered with warm sterile saline and the transducer is partially immersed in the fluid. The transducer is moved across the eye and the child may be asked to look in different directions. The echoes are displayed by B-mode on the oscilloscope screen, and the significant information is photographed.

When the necessary information has been obtained, the eyelid retractor is removed and the water bath is drained.

The drape is then removed, and the area around the eye is dried.

Preparation: No physical preparation is needed. The child and parents should be given a simple explanation of the procedure and its purpose. The child should be reassured that there will be no discomfort during the procedure. If general anesthesia is to be used, the child should be prepared accordingly.

Certain ophthalmic scanning instruments operate with the probe placed directly on the cornea or on the closed upper lid. Other scanning units require that the eye be immersed in a water bath for scanning. The child should be told which type of procedure will be performed so he will know what is expected of him. Special drops will be put in his eye before the examination so he will not feel the probe. Immersion of the eye in the water bath has been described as feeling strange but not uncomfortable. The child must understand the importance of lying quietly during the test. Younger or uncooperative children may be examined under general anesthesia.

Aftercare: If general anesthesia is used, the child is kept in the recovery room until he is awake and can take fluids. If only topical anesthesia is used, the child should be cautioned not to rub his eyes in order to protect the cornea from injury. In infants and younger children, elbow restraints may be necessary to prevent damage to the cornea. The topical anesthesia usually wears off in about 30 minutes. No attempt should be made to remove collodion from around the orbit until the topical anesthesia has worn off.

FLUORESCEIN ANGIOGRAPHY

Fluorescein angiography is an invasive procedure used to evaluate retinal and choroidal circulation. This procedure is valuable in documenting hemorrhage or fluid within the retinal tissue due to trauma, inflammation, or vascular abnormalities.

Premedication: Mydriatic cycloplegic eye drops are instilled before the examination to dilate the pupils. Cyclogyl drops are administered 30 to 40 minutes before the procedure, one drop in each eye, 5 minutes apart. When atropine ointment is the cycloplegic of choice, it is administered at home three times a day for two days before the examination.

Diet: No restriction is necessary.

Consent: An authorization signed by the parent or guardian is advisable.

Time: 1 hour.

Procedure: The pupils are dilated with mydriatic cycloplegic eye drops instilled two times within a 5-minute interval, 30 to 45 minutes before the examination. The room used for the study should be dark. The child is seated comfortably in an examination chair with his chin and forehead immobilized in a frame to facilitate correct focusing for the photographs. One arm is extended for injection, and fluorescein dye is injected into an antecubital vein over a 2- to 3-second period. The circulation of the eye is then carefully examined with an indirect opthalmoscope for the first 30 seconds, at 3 to 5 minutes, and at 20 to 60 minutes from the time of injection. Photographs documenting retinal and choroidal circulation are also taken at these intervals.

Preparation: No physical preparation is needed. The child and parents should be given a simple explanation of the procedure and its purpose. Eye drops will be instilled before the test to open the pupil as widely as possible. The drops may sting briefly and cause an unusual taste in the mouth. These sensations last only a few minutes. A waiting period of 30 to 45 minutes is necessary for adequate pupil dilation. A special medium (fluorescein) will be injected into the child's arm, and the physician will then look into the child's eyes with a machine that shines a bright light. The machine will also take pictures of the inside of the eye. The physician will look into the eye and take pictures immediately after the injection and then at 5, 10, and 60 minutes.

The major discomfort during the procedure is associated with venipuncture. Fluorescein toxicity is rare (incidence less than 1%). Reactions to fluorescein range from mild itching, erythema, and hives to anaphylactic reactions. (1). Transient nausea 15 to 20 seconds after injection occurs in about five percent of patients and seems to be associated with rapid injection (2). An emergency tray should be available when fluorescein is administered.

The child must understand the importance of remaining still during the study.

Restraint Necessary: The child may require restraint during the instillation of the eye drops and the injection of the dye, but proper explanation and reassurance should suffice for the remainder of the procedure.

Aftercare: Pupil dilation may cause the eyes to be extremely sensitive to bright light for a few hours. Wearing dark glasses may increase comfort. Near vision will be impaired until the effects of the eye drops have worn off. Fluorescein causes the urine to appear reddish for approximately 45 hours.

INDIRECT OPHTHALMOSCOPY

Indirect ophthalmoscopy is a noninvasive procedure that permits visualization of the posterior portion of the eye and is useful whenever ophthalmoscopic examination is indicated. The advantages of this method over direct ophthalmoscopy are *1*) the field of view is larger; *2*) there is more illumination; and *3*) the view is stereoscopic. In addition, the more remote position of the examiner provides easier access and may be less threatening to small children.

Premedication: Mydriatic cycloplegic eye drops are instilled before the examination to dilate the pupils. Cyclogyl drops are administered 30 to 40 minutes before the procedure, one drop in each eye, 5 minutes apart. The drops may sting briefly and cause an unusual taste in the mouth. These sensations last only a few minutes. Wben atropine ointment is the cycloplegic of choice, it is administered at home three times a day for two days before the examination.

Diet: No restriction is necessary.

Time: 15 to 30 minutes.

Procedure: The child may be sitting or supine in the darkened examination room. The ophthalmoscope worn on the examiner's head permits him to use both hands, one to hold the eye open and the other to hold a convex lens before the eye (Fig. 9-1). The hand-held lens focuses the light reflected from the retina into an inverted image seen by the examiner. The eyes are examined separately. The child is instructed to keep both eyes open and to look in various directions while the various segments of the retina are being examined.

Preparation: No physical preparation is needed. The child and parents should be given a simple explanation of the procedure and its purpose. It is essential that the child remain still during the examination. The physician will ask the child to keep both eyes open and to look in various directions during the test. The physician will be wearing an instrument on his head (a "moon hat"), which shines a

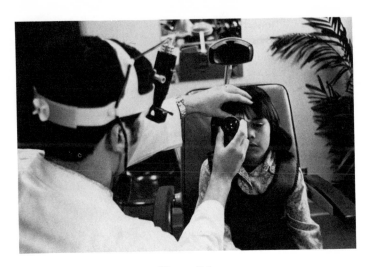

Figure 9-1
Indirect ophthalmoscopy.

bright light. He will hold a lens over the child's eye with one hand and hold the eyelid open with the other.

Restraint Necessary: Children under 2 years of age may require restraint. An effective method is to place the child on the parent's lap with his legs straddling the parent's waist, and his head held between the parent's knees. The child's hands can be held by the parent across his chest.

Aftercare: Pupil dilation may cause the eyes to be extremely sensitive to bright light for a few hours. Wearing dark glasses may increase comfort. Near vision will be impaired until the effects of the eye drops have worn off.

RETINOSCOPY

Retinoscopy (objective refraction) provides an objective method of determining refractive errors of the eye. The examiner projects light into the child's eyes and judges the error of refraction by the distortion of the reflected light rays. Retinoscopy is particularly valuable in pediatrics because it enables the examiner to measure refractive error without relying on the child's subjective responses.

Premedication: Mydriatic cycloplegic eye drops are instilled before examination to dilate the pupils. Cyclogyl drops are administered 30 to 40 minutes before the procedure, one drop in each eye, 5 minutes apart. The drops may sting briefly and cause an unusual taste in the mouth. These sensations last only a few minutes. When atropine ointment is the cycloplegic of choice, it is administered at home three times a day for two days before the examination.

Diet: No restriction is necessary.

Time: 15 to 30 minutes.

Procedure: The child is seated in an examination chair or on his mother's lap. The examiner holds the retinoscope approximately two feet from the child's eyes and observes the light reflex. Since the focus of light is characteristically distorted by refractive error, the examiner can objectively determine the refractive error of the eye. The child is asked to look directly at the light of the retinoscope. Lenses of varying strengths, hand held or mounted in spectacles or a Phoropter, are placed before the eyes during retinoscopy to determine tbe degree of correction required. Children old enough to respond to a visual acuity chart are asked to read successively smaller letters as the lenses are varied.

Preparation: No physical preparation is needed. The child and parents should be given a simple explanation of the procedure and its purpose. The child will sit in an examining chair and the examiner will look into his eyes with a bright light held in his hand. The child will wear special glasses during the test or will look through a machine. The child must remain still during the examination and look directly at the light of the retinoscope.

Aftercare: Pupil dilation may cause the eyes to be extremely sensitive to bright light for a few hours. Wearing dark glasses may increase comfort. Near vision will be impaired until the effects of the eye drops have worn off.

SLIT LAMP EXAMINATION

Slit lamp examination (biomicroscopy) is a noninvasive procedure that provides a highly magnified and well-illuminated view of the eye.

Premedication: Mydriatic cycloplegic eye drops are instilled before examination to dilate the pupils. Cyclogyl drops are administered 30 to 40 minutes before the procedure, one drop in each eye, 5 minutes apart. The drops may sting briefly and cause an unusual taste in the mouth. These sensations last only a few minutes. When atropine ointment is the cycloplegic of choice, it is administered at home three times a day for two days before the examination.

Time: 10 to 15 minutes.

Procedure: The child and the examiner are seated facing each other. Small children and infants usually respond best if they are seated on their mothers' laps. The child's chin is placed on a chin rest and his forehead is placed against a frame for immobilization (Fig. 9-2). If the child is old enough, he is instructed to look straight ahead without blinking. The examiner studies the eyes through the slit lamp while he moves the light source and the focus of the microscope back and forth.

Removal of foreign bodies, gonioscopy, or tonometry

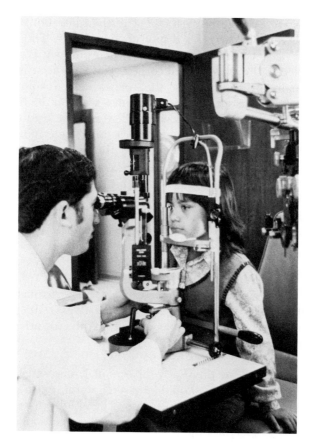

Figure 9-2
Slit lamp examination.

may be accomplished in older cooperative children during slit lamp examination after instillation of anesthetic eye drops.

Schiötz Tonometry: Tonometry provides a determination of intraocular pressure by measuring the degree of indentation that the tonometer plunger, which carries a fixed amount of weight, makes on the cornea. Anesthetic eye drops are instilled in each eye. The child lies on his back and is asked to stare at a spot on the ceiling. The tonometer, a metal instrument held by the examiner, is gently touched to the anesthetized cornea. The tonometer is then gradually pressed against the cornea, and readings of intraocular pressure are noted from a scale on the instrument. The greater the pressure, the lower the reading on the tonometer scale. Intraocular pressure is determined by referring to a chart that converts the scale readings in millimeters of mercury.

Gonioscopy: Gonioscopy is the examination of the angle of the anterior chamber. After instillation of anesthetic eye drops, a special type of contact lens device is applied to the cornea. The child is instructed to keep his eyes open and to look straight ahead. The examiner then carefully observes the eye through the slit lamp.

Both tonometry and gonioscopy can be performed under general anesthesia. Since all sedatives reduce the intraocular pressure, premedication, except for atropine, is usually avoided (1).

Preparation: No physical preparation is necessary. The child and his parents should be given a simple explanation of the procedure and its purpose. The child will rest his chin on the slit lamp frame while the physician looks into his eyes with a bright light. If other procedures are to be performed in conjunction with the slit lamp examination, anesthetic eye drops will be instilled to prevent discomfort. The child and parent should be forewarned if additional procedures are anticipated, and appropriate explanation should be provided.

Aftercare: If anesthetic eye drops were instilled, the child's cornea should be protected from trauma for 30 to 45 minutes, until the local anesthetic wears off and the protective reflexes return. The child's hands and other objects should be kept away from the eyes.

VISUAL ACUITY

Visual acuity may be evaluated with a number of different noninvasive tests, depending on the age of the child.

Premedication: None.

Diet: No dietary restriction necessary.

Time: 10 to 15 minutes, depending on the child's ability to cooperate.

Procedure: The measurement of visual acuity involves many factors unrelated to the ability to see test objects. Motivation, attention span, the patience of the examiner, and the child's fatigue or hunger all affect the accuracy of assessing visual acuity. Every effort should be made to control or minimize such variables. However, reasons for the child's unwillingness or inability to cooperate may be beyond the examiner's control, and several testing situations may be necessary to obtain valid results.

Visual acuity is measured in terms of the ability to see a standardized symbol at a standardized distance (3). Visual acuity is recorded as a combination of two numbers: the first indicates the distance to the chart, and the second indicates the distance at which a "normal" eye could read the line. Thus 20/40 means that the child is 20 feet from the chart and can read the line that a "normal" eye should see at 40 feet. The designation 20/40 is not a fraction and should not be interpreted as representing vision half as good as 20/20. Many authorities state that children do not develop 20/20 vision until after the age of 7 years. However, newer methods of evaluating visual acuity such as forced choice preferential looking (FPL) and visual evoked potential (VEP) have detected development of 20/20 acuity as early as 6 months of age.

Since the ability to respond appropriately to subjective

acuity tests (such as the Snellen test) requires mastery of such age related skills as the ability to recognize and name letters or pictures, concentration, and a relatively prolonged attention span, very young children do not perform as well on these tests as older children. Most authorities agree that children from the age of 4 to 7 years should be able to read the 20/30 line of the Snellen chart accurately with both eyes, and children younger than 4 years are expected to read the 20/40 line. Children 8 years old should be able to read the 20/20 line. The Snellen chart is used most often with children 8 years of age and older. The child is placed 20 feet from the chart and is tested as far down the chart as he is able to read. A passing score for a line consists of reading the majority of letters on that line (20/30 ±1). Although the acuity of each eye is measured separately, the test may be begun by testing both eyes at once to accustom the child to the procedure. An entire line or the whole chart should be exposed at once rather than a series of letters, especially in children with amblyopia. Even normal vision tested by the single letter method can appear up to one or two lines better than when tested by exposure of an entire line. The child's eyes should be covered carefully, preferably with an occluder of some type, to prevent "peeking." Also, pressure on the covered eye should be avoided or vision may be blurred after the eye is uncovered.

For children 3 years of age and older who are unable to read the alphabet chart, the Snellen "E" or "Illiterate E" may be used. These charts have the letter "E" oriented in four directions: up, down, right, and left. The child is asked to indicate which way the "E" is pointing. Unfortunately, this procedure evaluates not only vision, but otber complicated skills such as determination of direction and eye-hand coordination. To eliminate the problem of motor maneuvering, Brown (3) suggests pasting easily recognized pictures (e.g., dog, rabbit, boy, girl) on the wall at the top, bottom, and each side of the chart and then asking the child to tell to which picture the "E" is pointing.

The Stycar chart was developed in England and is now widely used in this country. The child holds in his lap a large card containing either five, seven, or nine different letters depending on the child's age and ability. He is asked to point to the letter on his card that matches the large test letter on the chart the examiner shows him. One eye is occluded, and he is asked to identify progressively smaller letters on the test chart 10 feet away.

Other commonly used letter tests include the Landholt rings, which uses the letter "C", and the Ffooks chart, which displays the geometric figures of a square, a circle, and a triangle. These tests have not been as accurate for pediatric testing as the Snellen charts (3).

Various picture charts are available, but these are less standardized and therefore less accurate than the letter tests mentioned above. Picture tests rely on the verbal achievement of the child to a large degree. For this reason, the child should be permitted to call a picture by any name so long as he is consistent. One of the most widely used of the picture tests is the Allen cards, which consists of a series of black and white pictures (e.g., telephone, man, horse, Christmas tree, birthday cake, etc.). The cards are shown to the child by an examiner who slowly moves toward the child. The distance at which the child is able to recognize three of the pictures is used as the numerator over a denominator of 30. Acceptable scores are 15/30 for 3 year olds and 20/30 for 4 year olds (3).

Other picture charts available are the Osterberg chart, a black and white chart of figures (swan, Christmas tree, house, tree, man, and key); the kindergarten chart, with color pictures of a circle, cross, heart, flag, and sailboat; the A.O. and B & L tests which have similar pictures in black and white; and the California clown test, in which a clown's hand points in different directions.

Many children, especially those with amblyopia, attempt to peek around whatever is occluding the good eye. For this reason, the child should not be asked to hold the occluder himself.

In small infants, detection of optokinetic nystagmus* is used to measure visual acuity. Optokinetic targets, such as a tape measure or a strip of cloth with 2-inch color squares sewn 2 inches apart or a rotating drum covered with red and white stripes or brightly colored pictures, are passed before the infant's eyes to elicit optokinetic nystagmus. The optokinetic (OKN) response may be assessed by the examiner or recorded on a polygraph. The test indicates intact cortical visual responses, but gives only a rough estimate of acuity. Ability to fix and follow a light, generally present by 2 months of age and well established by 3 months, is also assessed (1).

An essential part of the eye examination is testing for alignment of the eyes to detect strabismus or nonbinocular vision. Strabismus is a disorder in which both eyes cannot fix on one object simultaneously due to a lack of muscular coordination. Usually strabismus can be corrected by patching and/or corrective lenses if it is detected early. But if it is left untreated until the age of 4 to 6 years, the visual acuity in the misaligned eye (amblyopia) may become worse. Because of the risk of a permanent visual deviation, strabismus should be corrected as early as possible.

Two techniques useful in detecting strabismus are the corneal light reflex test and the cover test. In the corneal light reflex test (Hirschberg's reflex test) the child is asked to look straight ahead while the examiner shines a pen light directly into the child's eyes from a distance of about 16 inches. The light reflection in each pupil should be in the exact same position. If the light is even slightly off-center in one eye, strabismus is present. The inward

*Keltner describes optokinetic nystagmus as "the involuntary rhythmic oscillation of the eyes produced by a repetitive stimulus passing in front of the child's visual field. There is a slow phase as the eyes follow one target and then a corrective fast phase as they shift to pick up the next target coming into view. The phenomenon has been called 'railroad train nystagmus,' from the well-known example of the passenger on a moving train who glances out the window and focuses on each telephone pole as it comes into view" (4).

deviation of the eye is called esotropia or esophoria; the outward deviation is called exotropia or exophoria. A tropia (overt strabismus) is a condition in which the eyes are not aligned for binocular viewing. A child with a tropia frequently manifests an apparent deviation ("cross-eye"). A phoria is a tendency for one eye to drift out of proper alignment, especially when one eye is covered. A child with a phoria may be able to keep his eyes straight by exerting effort to maintain fusion, resulting in eyestrain.

In the cover test the child is asked to focus on an object about 12 inches from his eyes. The child is encouraged to look steadily at the object and to keep both eyes open. The examiner then occludes the vision of one eye and watches for movement of the uncovered eye. If the uncovered eye moves, some degree of strabismus is present. The cover test is repeated with the child focusing on a distant object. Both eyes should be tested.

In the alternate cover test the occluder is moved directly from one eye to the other without allowing binocular viewing. If movement of either eye occurs, a phoria is present.

Steropsis, the ability to see well in three dimensions at close range, is tested with the Titmus (or Wirt) stereo test. The child views a hand-held booklet while wearing Polaroid spectacles ("magic glasses"). The first picture in the booklet consists of an enlarged stereo photograph of a housefly. The child with normal binocular vision is able to successfully fuse the stereogram and see a three-dimensional "monster" fly (15 cm × 10 cm) standing out from the booklet by about 5 cm. A child using only one eye cannot fuse the stereogram and sees only a flat, two-dimensional picture of a fly. Children with strabismus often suppress vision of one eye and therefore do not have stereopsis. Suppression of one eye can be detected with the Worth four dots test. The child wears special glasses with a red lens before one eye and a green lens before the other. Red, green, and white colored lights are presented to the child through a flashlight test instrument or a display box at a specified distance. The child is asked to tell what colors he sees when the lights are presented.

A number of screening tools are available for assessing color vision. The Hardy-Rand-Rittler (HRR) pseudoiso-chromatic plates are included in a booklet of 24 pictures of gray versus color-confusable dots. The dots are set in patterns, all of which are recognizable to the person with normal color vision. A color-blind person is unable to identify the various forms on the plates. The first pictures demonstrate, even to the child with color-defective vision, the three forms of colored test figures (a circle, an X, and a triangle) immersed within a field pattern of gray dots. The remaining plates evaluate defects in color vision. The Ishihara test is an even more exact screen that no one with a color defect can read without making some mistakes (2). The Farnsworth D-15 color chips may be used for children who fail the HRR or Ishihara tests. A reference chip of color is presented to the child along with 15 movable chips of hue progression. The child is asked to arrange the 15 chips in order of progression. This test is simple, inexpensive, and can be easily accomplished by most children over 4 years of age. The Farnsworth D-15 is not as discriminating as the two former tests. Only significant color defectives fail the color chip test.

Peripheral vision is evaluated by asking the child to gaze straight ahead and indicate in which portion of the peripheral field the examiner's finger is wiggling. For infants and very young children, the parent is asked to create a distraction while a bright (noiseless) object is moved into the peripheral field from behind. Response to the object indicates adequate peripheral vision.

Preparation: Since visual acuity tests require that the child identify certain letters or pictures, practice before the examination is helpful. A particularly useful method is to ask the mother to practice with the child at home during the week before the test. The National Society for Prevention of Blindness has "E" charts available at no cost for practice testing at home. Such practice improves the child's cooperation and increases the accuracy of the test.

REFERENCES

1. Harley RD: *Pediatric Ophthalmology.* Philadelphia, WB Saunders Co, 1975.
2. Keeney AH: *Ocular Examination,* ed 2. St Louis, CV Mosby Co, 1976.
3. Brown MS: Vision Screening of Preschool Children. *Clin Pediatr* 14(10):968, 1975.
4. Keltner JL: Neuro-opthalmology for the Pediatrician. *Pediatr Ann* 6(2):78, 1977.

BIBLIOGRAPHY

Brant JC, Nowotny M: Testing of Visual Acuity in Young Children: An Evaluation of Some Commonly Used Methods. *Dev Med Child Neurol* 18:568, 1976.

Brown MS: Vision Screening of Preschool Children. *Clin Pediatr* 14(10):968, 1975.

Harden A: Non-corneal electroretinogram. *Br J Ophthalmol* 58:811, 1974.

Harrison A: Methods of Assessing Visual Acuity in Young Children. *Am Orthoptic J* 25:109, 1975.

Keeney AH: *Ocular Examination,* ed 2. St Louis, CV Mosby Co, 1976.

Keltner JL: Neuro-ophthalmology for the Pediatrician. *Pediatr Ann* 6(2):78, 1977.

McCrary JA: *Pediatric Oculo-Neural Diseases.* Flushing, NY, Medical Examining Publishing Co, 1973.

Moody EM, Gibson G: Ophthalmic Examination of Infants and Children, in Harley RD (ed): *Pediatric Ophthalmology.* Philadelphia, WB Saunders Co, 1975, p 59.

Newell FW, Ernest JT: *Ophthalmology,* ed 3. St Louis, CV Mosby Co, 1974.

Saunders WH, Havener WH, Fair CJ, et al: *Nursing Care in Eyes, Ear, Nose and Throat Disorders.* St Louis, CV Mosby Co, 1968.

Scipien GM, Barnard MU, Chard MA, et al: *Comprehensive Pediatric Nursing.* McGraw-Hill Book Co, 1975.

Sorsby A: *Modern Ophthalmology,* Vol 1, ed 2. Philadelphia JB Lippincott Co, 1972.

Stager DR: Amblyopia and the Physician. *Pediatr Ann* 6(2):46, 1977.

Vaughan D, Asbury T, Cook R: *General Ophthalmology.* Los Altos, Ca, Lange Medical Publications, 1971.

10

Ultrasound Procedures

ULTRASONOGRAPHY

Ultrasound is a valuable noninvasive diagnostic tool that can make a significant contribution to the investigation of numerous pediatric conditions.

Ultrasonography is based on the same principle as the oceanographic technique of sonar (sound navigation ranging). Pulsing sound waves with frequencies that are too high to be detected by the human ear* are emitted by a transducer. These sound waves travel through the tissues and their echoes are reflected back to the transducer, which also functions as a receiver. The transducer is made of a piezoelectric substance that converts electric impulses into ultrasound waves and then reconverts the returning echoes to electricity. A large margin of safety exists since the piezoelectric crystal sends pulses for only 0.1% of the time and receives for 99.9% of the time (4). The returning echoes can be displayed in a number of ways. In the A-mode (amplitude modulated) scan, the echo information is displayed by vertical lines on an oscilloscope that represent the relative strength of the echoes. A-mode provides a one-dimensional display. B-mode (brightness modulated) is two-dimensional and displays echoes as dots instead of vertical lines. As a result, the oscilloscope reveals a series of dots whose brightness represents the amplitude of the

---

*Ultrasound is a frequency range above 20,000 cycles/second or hertz (Hz). Medical ultrasound is currently confined to frequencies between 1 and 10 megahertz (MHz). This safety margin prevents the possibility of heat production or cavitation (4). Ultrasound at these diagnostic frequencies has no known deleterious side-effects.

echo and whose position identifies the distances of the reflecting structures below the transducer (5). M-mode (time-motion) is useful for studying moving structures such as the heart. The M-mode is simply a type of B-mode display in which the oscilloscope picture is allowed to build up progressively from the X-axis. The results are recorded on Polaroid film or on a strip chart recorder.

Recently, a technique has been developed that displays the echo in the form of a shaded picture, the gray scale display. This modality reveals the texture and boundaries of certain structures more clearly than other modes. Information may be recorded either with photographic film or with a scan conversion memory, which can display the stored image continuously on a standard television monitor (5).

Sound waves travel more easily through solids than through liquid or gaseous media. Air in the lungs or gas in the bowel present a barrier to ultrasound examinations (6). Various anatomic "windows" must often be used, for example, along the sternal border for cardiac scanning. For the same reason, mineral oil or a commercial gel is applied to provide an airless contact between the transducer and the skin. Bone either reflects or absorbs the ultrasonic energy that strikes it, so the waves must be directed about bony structures as well as around gas-filled ones (7).

Since ultrasound is painless and the time required for examination is short, usually no premedication is necessary. The procedure is so innocuous that many children sleep throughout the examination.

ABDOMINAL ULTRASONOGRAPHY

Ultrasonography of the abdomen is useful in the detection of space-occupying lesions of the abdomen, liver, and pancreas or of retroperitoneal nodes over 2 cm in size.

Probably the most effective application of abdominal ul-trasonography is in the evaluation of renal pathology. Ultrasound also provides a simple, noninvasive method of assessing residual urine in the bladder. Aspiration biopsy of liver lesions under diagnostic ultrasound control, using a special transducer with a central hole through which a biopsy needle is passed, has been reported to increase accuracy of the procedure (1). Suprapubic bladder aspi-ration using the same technique has also been advocated (1,2).

Premedication: None.

Diet: No restriction is necessary unless the gallbladder is to be examined, in which case the child should be kept NPO overnight.

Time: 15 minutes.

Procedure: The child is placed in a supine position and mineral oil or a water-soluble gel is applied to the abdo-men. In older children, the prone position may be used to visualize the kidneys, in which case gel is applied to the lower back. The transducer is placed firmly over the prepared area and is passed horizontally across the child's abdomen or back at 1- or 2-cm intervals. The echoes are displayed by B-mode on the oscilloscope and significant information is recorded on photographic paper or film.

After the necessary information has been obtained, the transducer is removed and the gel is washed off the child's skin.

Preparation: No physical preparation is needed. The child and parents should be given a simple explanation of the procedure and its purpose. A small amount of oil or gel will be applied to the child's abdomen. Then a small instrument, the transducer, will be placed firmly over the area and moved back and forth for a few minutes. The child will feel a slight pressure or a tickling sensation from the transducer. The child should understand the importance of remaining still during the procedure.

Aftercare: No physical aftercare is necessary.

ECHOCARDIOGRAPHY

Echocardiography provides recordings of the motion of the mitral, aortic, tricuspid, and pulmonic valves, the interventricular septum and the right and left ventricular walls. It also reveals the size of the cardiac chambers and the changes of these dimensions during the cardiac cycle (3). Such information is valuable for diagnosing congenital heart disease, for assessing the results of cardiac surgery, or for determining the timing of cardiac catheterization.

Premedication: None.

Diet: No restriction necessary.

Time: 15 to 30 minutes.

Procedure: The child is placed in a supine position on the examination table or in bed. A water-soluble gel or mineral oil is applied to the skin of the chest wall and to the face of the transducer. The transducer is placed firmly on the chest wall so that it is in complete contact and is moved back and forth in various directions and at different angles (Fig. 10-1). The ultrasonic window, which extends along the left sternal border and somewhat toward the apex of the heart, is used to avoid interference from the lung. The echocardiogram, displayed by M-mode, is recorded on photographic paper (strip chart recording) or on Polaroid film.

When the necessary information has been obtained, the transducer is removed and the gel is washed off the child's skin.

Preparation: No physical preparation is needed. The child and parents should be given a simple explanation of the procedure and its purpose. A small amount of oil or gel will be applied to the skin on the child's chest. An instrument, a transducer, will be placed firmly on the chest and is moved back and forth. The child will experience no discomfort during the procedure. The child must understand the necessity of holding still during the procedure.

Aftercare: No physical aftercare is necessary.

ECHOENCEPHALOGRAPHY

Echoencephalography is useful in identifying supratento-

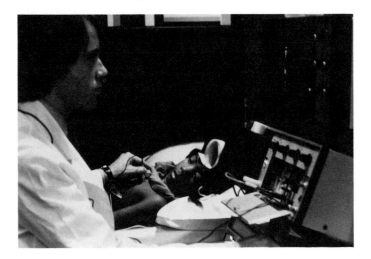

Figure 10-1
Echocardiography.

rial masses by measuring the position of structures in the cerebral midline. The distance from the skull to the third ventricle is measured on each side. Because the third ventricle should be in the exact center of the brain, this test reveals if there is anything displacing one side of the brain (e.g., intracranial hematoma or tumor).

Premedication: None.

Diet: No restriction necessary.

Time: 10 minutes.

Procedure: The child is placed in a sitting or supine position and mineral oil or a water soluble gel is applied just above the fleshy part of both ears. Two transducers are placed firmly over the gel to form an air-tight seal. The diameter of the head is thus determined. Then a single transducer is placed first over one ear and then the other to determine the position of the midline structure. The echoes are displayed by A-mode on the oscilloscope screen and significant information is photographed.

   After the necessary information has been obtained, the transducers are removed and the gel is washed off the child's skin.

Preparation: No physical preparation is needed. The child and parents should be given a simple explanation of the procedure and its purpose. A small amount of oil or gel will be applied to the skin on the child's head above his ears. Two small instruments, transducers, will be placed firmly on these areas for a few minutes and then removed. The child will experience no discomfort during the procedure. The child must understand the necessity of holding still during the procedure.

Aftercare: No physical aftercare is necessary.

REFERENCES

1. James AE, Wagner HN, Cooke RE: *Pediatr Nuclear Medicine.* Philadelphia WB Saunders Co, 1974.
2. Goldberg BB, Pollack HM, Capitanio MA, et al: Ultrasonography: An Aid in the Diagnosis of Masses in Pediatric Patients. *Pediatrics* 56(3):421, 1975.
3. Tilkian SM, Conover MH: *Clinical Implications of Laboratory Tests.* St. Louis, CV Mosby Co, 1975.
4. Dempsey PJ: The Role of Abdominal Sonography in Pediatric Diagnosis. *Pediatr Ann* 5(1):103, 1976.
5. Bronzino JP: *Technology for Patient Care.* St Louis, CV Mosby Co, 1977.
6. Carlsen EN: Ultrasound Physics for the Physician, A Brief Review. *J Clin Ultrasound* 3(1):69, 1975.
7. Coats K: Non-Invasive Cardiac Diagnostic Procedures. *Am J Nurs* 75(11):1980, 1975.

BIBLIOGRAPHY

Bronzino JD: *Technology for Patient Care.* St Louis, CV Mosby Co, 1977.

Brown B, Gordon D (eds): *Ultrasonic Techniques in Biology and Medicine* Springfield, Ill, Charles C Thomas, 1967.

Buddemeyer EU: The Physics of Diagnostic Ultrasound. *Radiol Clin North Am* 13(3):391, 1975.

Carlsen EN: Ultrasound Physics for the Physician, A Brief Review. *J Clin Ultrasound* 3(1):69, 1975.

Coats K: Non-Invasive Cardiac Diagnostic Procedures. *Am J Nurs* 75(11): 1980, 1975.

Dempsey PJ: The Role of Abdominal Sonography in Pediatric Diagnosis. *Pediatr Ann* 5(1):103, 1976.

Goldberg BB (ed): *Abdominal Gray Scale Ultrasonography.* New York, John Wiley & Sons, 1977.

Goldberg BB, Pollack HM, Capitanio MA, et al: Ultrasonography: An Aid in the Diagnosis of Masses in Pediatric Patients. *Pediatrics* 56(3):421, 1975.

Harrison SW, Parks C, Sherwood T: Ultrasound Assessment of Residual Urine in Children. *Br J Urol* 47(7):805, 1976.

James AE, Wagner HN, Cooke RE: *Pediatr Nuclear Medicine.* Philadelphia, WB Saunders Co, 1974.

Lippe BM, Sample FW: Pelvic Ultrasonography in Pediatric and Adolescent Endocrine Disorders. *J Pediatr* 92(6):897, 1978.

Rocha AF, Harbert JC: *Textbook of Nuclear Medicine: Basic Science.* Philadelphia, Lea & Febiger, 1978.

Saunders RC: B-Scan Ultrasound in the Management of Abdominal Masses in Children. *JAMA* 231(1):81, 1975.

Tilkian SM, Conover MH: *Clinical Implications of Laboratory Tests.* St Louis, CV Mosby Co, 1975.

11

Radionuclide Diagnostic Procedures

In recent years the use of radioactive materials to provide diagnostic information has increased at a phenomenal rate. Radionuclides can be used as tracers within the body (in vivo tests) or in body fluids that have been removed from the patient (in vitro tests). In vivo radionuclide studies require patient preparation and cooperation. These studies will be the focus of this section's discussion.

Radiopharmaceuticals are radionuclides or radioactive-labeled elements whose physical properties enable them to concentrate selectively in a target organ or system that is being studied. For most organs (kidney, liver, lung), the radiopharmaceutical concentrates in normal functioning tissue, and the diseased areas are visualized as areas of decreased activity. In a few organ systems, however (brain and bone), abnormal tissue concentrates the radiopharmaceutical to a greater degree than normal tissue. Physical properties considered in choosing radiopharmaceuticals include the type of radiations emitted, the energy of the radiations, and the half-life. In children, the radiation dose must be as small as possible while providing the necessary diagnostic information. Radionuclides used in diagnostic studies emit gamma radiation. For in vitro studies, half-lives of a few days to a few months are acceptable. For internal administration, short half-life radionuclides are best, since the shorter the half-life, the less the radiation dose to the patient per millicurie (mC:). The most desirable half-life for in vivo studies is a few hours to a few days. The short biologic half-lives and the minute amounts used for in vivo studies make the radiation hazard of the radiopharmaceuticals negligible. The amount of radiation emitted by such radiopharmaceuticals is so small that usually no special precautions are necessary in handling the child or his excreta after the procedure.

Examples of commonly used radionuclides are ^{99m}Tc pertechnetate and iodine 123 (^{123}I).

Radiation that is emitted by the radionuclide is detected and measured by either a retilinear scanner or a gamma camera, which work on the same basic principle. A photoelectric cell within the system detects the radiation, and a flash of light is produced when each gamma photon strikes the scintillation crystal. The light flashes are converted within a photomultiplier tube into electric pulses that are amplified and then recorded. The scintillation output data are processed through an imaging device that displays the area under study on photographic film, x-ray film, or on a television screen. Some imaging devices provide a color display of detected radiation.

The rectilinear scanner, possessing a single crystal, has a very small field of view and must be moved back and forth across the organ (in one or more planes) until the area has been completely surveyed by the scintillation detector. Rectilinear scanners are very rarely used in pediatrics today, since they generally take a considerable amount of time to build an image of the patient. The gama camera, or scintillation camera, builds up an image more quickly than the retilinear scanner and, with proper collimators, provides excellent resolution. The gamma camera remains stationary instead of moving back and forth; its numerous scintillation crystals provide a large field of vision encompassing all parts of the radiation field continuously. The image produced by the gamma camera is viewed on an oscilloscope screen and may be recorded on file or on digital tape for dynamic studies. The data collected can also be supplied to a computer for further processing and image enhancement.

BONE SCAN

Bone scanning is a noninvasive nuclear imaging procedure useful in the diagnosis of skeletal disease. Indications for bone scanning include evaluation for bone tumor or bony metastatic disease and evaluation for early osteomyelitis or fractures not visualized on x-ray film (1). Bone scanning is a sensitive indicator of bone disease at a very early stage before it is detectable radiographically.

Premedication: If technetium (^{99m}Tc) is to be used, a blocking agent is administered 1 hour before the injection of the radionuclide. (refer to Table 11-1).

Diet: No dietary restriction is necessary.

Consent: An authorization signed by the parent or guardian is necessary.

Time: 1 hour.

Procedure: The radiopharmaceutical, usually a ^{99m}Tc-labeled compound, is injected intravenously 3 hours before the scan (refer to Table 11-1). The child is encouraged to drink fluids during the waiting period.

The child is placed under the scanner (the position depends on the area to be studied) and images are obtained.

Preparation: (See section on "Brain Scan.") The child should drink as much water as possible after the injection of the radiopharmaceutical to reduce the scatter and to promote renal excretion. The radionuclides used in pediatric bone scanning, ^{99m}Tc phosphates, are excreted pri-

Table 11-1
Radiopharmaceuticals Used in Brain Scanning

Procedure	Radio-nuclide	Form	Half-life	Time Lapse until Scan (Optimal)	Prior Preparation	Purpose of Blocking Agent	Principal Route of Elimination
Brain scan Bone scan Angiogram Lung scan	^{99m}Tc	Technetium pertechnetate	6 hours	30–60 minute 0–5 minute (Av abnormalities)	Oral: Potassium thiocyanate or potassium perchlorate 1 hour before injection of radionuclide	To block uptake by thyroid, choroid plexus, and salivary glands	Urine
Renal imaging						To block salivary gland to prevent artifact on scan	
Thyroid studies					Atropine (sometimes)		

Procedure	Radionuclide	Form	Half-life	Time of imaging	Preparation	Rationale	Route of excretion
Angiogram Cisternography Lung scan	^{99m}Tc	Human serum albumin	6 hours	2 – 3 hours 24 hours (late)			Urine
Liver scan	^{131}I	Iodinated human serum albumin	8.1 days	24 – 48 hours	Oral Lugol's solution daily for 1 day before injection of radionuclide and twice a day for a week after study[a]	To inhibit uptake by the thyroid	
Cisternography Thyroid studies	(Rarely used) ^{123}I		13.3 hours	2 hours	None	None	Urine
Lung scan	^{133}Xe	Xenon gas	5.27 days	10 – 15 seconds	None	None	Lungs

SOURCE: Adapted with permission from Mandrillo, M., Brain scanning. *Nurs. Clinics of N. Amer.* 9(4):633, December 1974.

[a]Excess iodide may cause vomiting in infants after administration for several days.

231

marily by the kidney. The bladder must be emptied immediately before the scan to visualize the pelvis adequately (1).

Restraint Necessary: (See section on "Brain Scan.")

Aftercare: No physical aftercare is necessary.

BRAIN SCAN

Brain scanning, the most frequently performed pediatric nuclear imaging procedure, provides a safe noninvasive screening technique that is generally used before resorting to contrast studies. Brain scanning is a valuable diagnostic tool performed on children who have seizures or other neurologic symptoms that could indicate a central nervous system disease.

Premedication: In most institutions, children are not routinely sedated before nuclear medicine procedures. Most camera images require only a few minutes and usually restraint is sufficient. Depending on the radiopharmaceutical chosen, a blocking agent may be administered 1 hour before the injection of the radionuclide (refer to Table 11-1).

Diet: If the child is not sedated, no dietary restriction is necessary.

Consent: An authorization signed by the parent or guardian is necessary.

Time: Rectilinear scanner; 45 to 60 minutes (seldom used). Gamma camera. 10 to 15 minutes.

Procedure: The radionuclide is injected intravenously by
a trained technician. Scalp veins are not used in infants
since infiltration of the radiopharmaceutical may stimulate
the appearance of a subdural effusion. The child is restrained as necessary and placed in a supine position
under the scanner or camera. At the designated optimal
time of absorption and concentration of the radiopharmaceutical, multiple imaging views are obtained (refer to
Table 11-1). Views, including frontal, posterior, vertex,
and both lateral views, are recorded. Delayed imaging 2
hours after injection is often performed. Early scans (5 to
10 minutes after injection) provide useful information
concerning dynamic cerebral blood flow. Late scans may
define alterations in blood brain permeability. Although
the mechanism by which radiopharmaceuticals accumulate
in abnormal tissue is not completely understood, it is
generally agreed that an alteration of the blood-brain
barrier is involved (1). Normal brain tissue does not allow
passage of radionuclides from the plasma. Under abnormal conditions, this selective permeability is disrupted and
the radionuclides pass into the area of diseased tissue (2).

Either a scintillation camera (gamma camera) or rectilinear scanner can be used for pediatric brain scanning.
Rectilinear scanning may be more sensitive in the detection
of deeper lesions, whereas the gamma camera better
indicates superficial lesions. The gamma camera is usually
preferable in pediatric patients because it is much more
rapid, thus reducing movement artifacts.

Preparation: The child and parents should be given an
explanation of the procedure. As advance preparation,
the child may or may not receive a blocking agent by
mouth or injection, depending on the radioisotope used.
A sedative may also be given. The child and parents
should be reassured that the scan is simple, safe, and
painless. The amount of radioactive agent used is so small
that there is no radiation hazard to the child or to the
people around him.

A technician will inject the radionuclide into the child's vein and then will remove the needle.

The child will lie on a table while a special camera takes pictures of where the radioactive drug is in his body.

The child should understand the importance of remaining absolutely still while the pictures are being taken. Straps or sandbags may be placed around the child's head and body to help him hold still. The scanner does not emit radiation; it only detects the radiation given off by the radiopharmaceutical.

Depending on the radiopharmaceutical chosen, a blocking agent may be administered to prevent uptake of the radionuclide by structures other than those under study (refer to Table 11-1). If technetium is used, an oral dose of potassium perchlorate or potassium thiocyanate is administered. This will block the uptake of technetium by the thyroid, choroid plexus, and salivary glands. Atropine is sometimes given to decrease saliva and tears containing radioactivity that may produce artifacts on the scan. Potassium perchlorate is not easily dissolved in water and may be more palatable in a flavored syrup.

Restraint Necessary: The child must remain still during brain scanning to prevent movement artifacts. Proper preparation, reassurance, and adequate restraint are essential.

Aftercare: No physical aftercare is necessary.

CISTERNOGRAPHY

Cisternography is an invasive nuclear imaging procedure in which a radionuclide is injected into the subarachnoid space, providing a sensitive indicator of altered formation, flow, and reabsorption of cerebrospinal fluid (CSF). Cisternography is useful in the evaluation of hydrocephalus, determination of potency of CSF diversionary shunts, assessment of abnormalities of CSF flow, and identification of CSF leak.

Premedication: Many infants and young children do not require premedication for cisternography. If sedation is required, it should be given intramuscularly 30 to 45 minutes before the procedure. Depending on the radiopharmaceutical chosen, a blocking agent may be administered 1 hour before the injection of the radionuclide (refer to Table 11-1).

Diet: The sedated child should be kept NPO 4 hours before the procedure to prevent possible vomiting and aspiration of gastric contents. If the child is not sedated, no dietary restriction is necessary.

Consent: An authorization signed by the parent or guardian is necessary.

Time: 10 to 15 minutes for lumbar puncture and injection of radionuclide.

1- to 3-hour interval before the scan.

45 to 60 minutes scanning with rectilinear scanner (rarely used).

10 to 15 minutes scanning with a gamma camera.

Images may be obtained at ½-, 1-, 4-, 24-, and 48-hour intervals after injection of the radionuclide.

Procedure: A lumbar puncture is performed, free CSF flow is assured, and the radiopharmaceutical is injected into the subarachnoid space. Unnecessary manipulation of the needle (such as for pressure measurements) is avoided to minimize epidural extravasation. The radiopharmaceutical Yb-169 is commonly used for CSF imaging.

One to 2 hours after the injection, the child is placed in a supine position under the scanner or camera and images are obtained at appropriate time intervals. Intervals of ½ hour, 1 hour, 6 hours, 24 hours, and 48 hours are common. Occasionally, imaging may be begun immediately after the injection for shunt patency evaluation. Anterior and lateral views are taken. The child should remain recumbent for the first few hours of the study to prevent extravasation at the injection site.

If a CSF leak is suspected, sterile cotton pledgets are placed in the nasopharynx and ears. The pledgets are removed and replaced, and their radioactivity is measured serially over several hours. If a leak is confirmed, a larger dose of radionuclide is injected by lumbar puncture. The child is placed in a supine position for 3 hours to prevent leakage and to allow time for the radionuclide to rise to the brain. After 3 to 4 hours, the patient is placed in a head-down position and scanning is performed with a gamma camera. The child may be asked to hold his breath and bear down (Valsalva maneuver) to encourage leakage during the scan.

Preparation: (Refer to sections on "Lumbar Puncture" and "Brain Scan.") Cisternography should be performed before pneumoencephalography or at least a week after it.

Restraint Necessary: (See sections on "Lumbar Puncture" and "Brain Scan.")

Aftercare: (See section on "Lumbar Puncture.") Temperature should be monitored closely for 24 hours; a fever may be an indication of meningitis. Bacterial meningitis may follow a CSF leak, and aseptic meningitis is a possible side effect when ^{131}I human serum albumin is used for cisternography.

LIVER SCAN

A liver scan is a noninvasive nuclear imaging procedure that provides information about both liver structure (e.g., size, shape, and location) and liver function (e.g., biliary duct patency).

Premedication: Depending on the radiopharmaceutical chosen, a blocking agent may be administered 1 hour before the injection of the radionuclide (refer to Table 11-1).

Diet: The child is kept NPO for 4 to 6 hours before the liver function scan.

Consent: An authorization signed by the parent or guardian is necessary.

Time:
Liver structure scan: 30 minutes.

Liver Function Scan (Rose Bengal Test): Up to four scans of approximately 30 minutes each within 24 hours. Additional scans at 24 and 48 hours may be required.

Procedure:

Liver Structure Scan: The radiopharmaceutical is injected intravenously and the child is placed supine for imaging. Imaging is started 10 to 15 minutes after administration of radiocolloid (e.g., ^{99m}Tc sulfur colloid) or 20 to 30 minutes after ^{131}I rose bengal. Anterior, posterior, and right and left lateral views are obtained. Either a rectilinear scanner or, more frequently, a gamma camera may be used for the liver structure scan.

Liver Function Scan: Rose bengal dye tagged with radioactive iodine is accumulated by the liver, excreted into tbe
bile, stored in the gallbladder, and then excreted into the
intestines. The scanning of this radioactive material indicates the effectiveness of hepatic function as well as patency of the biliary tree.

The ^{131}I rose bengal is injected intravenously. A small
amount of nonradioactive rose bengal is injected at the
same time to slow down excretion of the radioactive rose
bengal and to stabilize the counting rate. Scanning is
begun immediately after injection in order to observe the
uptake in the liver. In the healthy patient the gallbladder
can be visualized at approximately 20 minutes and intestinal excretion can be noted between 30 and 60 minutes.
At least two views, anterior and right lateral, are obtained.
If an obstruction is noted, sequential scans are performed
during a 24- to 48-hour period (3). Absence of radioactivity
in the bowel indicates biliary obstruction. In some institutions the child is given a fatty meal after the initial scan to
stimulate gallbladder contraction.

Blood clearance of rose bengal may also be measured
for differentiation between medical and surgical jaundice.
Three to 5 ml of heparinized blood samples are obtained
5 minutes and 20 minutes after the injection of ^{131}I rose
bengal. The percent of blood retention of the dye is then
calculated. The scanner is positioned over a nonhepatic
blood pool (e.g., the head) and the counts are recorded
for 30 minutes. The 5- and 20-minute counts are used for
the calculation of clearance (4).

Preparation: (See section on "Brain Scan.") If ^{131}I-labeled
aggregated human serum albumin or ^{131}I rose bengal is
used, Lugol's solution must be given to block the uptake
by the thyroid gland. The liver scan should precede any
type of barium study, since the barium in the colon could
interfere with the liver scan and lead to false-positive
results (3).

Restraint Necessary: (See section on "Brain Scan.")

Aftercare: If ^{131}I was used, oral Lugol's solution is administered twice a day for a week after the study.

LUNG SCAN

Lung scanning is a noninvasive nuclear imaging procedure that provides information about regional blood flow and ventilation. This simple procedure can be performed in any age group, including the premature infant (4).

Premedication: Usually none. Very young or uncooperative children may require sedation for tbe ventilatory lung scan.

Diet: The sedated child should be kept NPO for 4 hours to prevent possible vomiting and aspiration of gastric contents.

Consent: An authorization signed by the parent or guardian is necessary.

Time:

Gamma Camera Perfusion Scan: 20 minutes.

Gamma Camera Ventilatory Scan: 10 minutes.

Rectilinear Scanner: 1 hour (rarely used).

Procedure:

Perfusion Scan: A radiopharmaceutical (usually ^{99m}Tc-macroaggregated albumin, MAA, or ^{133}Xe in solution) is injected intravenously. The radionuclide particles lodge in precapillary arterioles, revealing pulmonary perfusion on the scan. The distribution of radioactivity reveals the pattern of blood flowing through the lungs. Gravity affects the regional distribution of blood flow in the lung. When the child is in a supine position, blood pressure becomes equal in all lung regions and the distribution of blood flow becomes uniform (5). Therefore, the child is placed in a supine position during injection of the radiopharmaceutical.

Scanning is begun immediately after the injection. A gamma camera is used for the perfusion scan. Four views are usually obtained: anterior, posterior, and right and left lateral.

Ventilatory Scan: The child breathes radioactive gas (oxygen and Xenon-133) through a closed system utilizing a mouthpiece and nose clip. Very young children may require sedation for use of a mask (1). Care must be taken to maintain a closed system to prevent room contamination and excessive radiation exposure.

Scanning is begun immediately as the child breathes the radioactive gas, which enters various regions of the lung at a rate directly related to the ventilation (5). Either a rectilinear scanner or a gamma camera may be used for the ventilatory scan, but the gamma camera's speed provides a definite advantage in children.

Preparation: (See section on "Brain Scan.") The child will breathe a special gas through a mouthpiece with nose clips in place or through a mask during part of the test. This gas will not make the child feel sleepy or unusual in any way. Practice sessions before the scan, breathing through the mouth with the nostrils held closed, are helpful.

The only discomfort involved in the test is during intravenous injection of the radiopharmaceutical.

Aftercare: If the child coughs productively, the sputum should be disposed of in a closed plastic container. The child may be given a drink of water after nebulization to ensure that no radioactive particles remain in the esophagus.

RADIONUCLIDE ANGIOCARDIOGRAPHY

Radionuclide angiocardiography is a noninvasive nuclear procedure that permits visualization of the course of blood flow through the heart. This procedure may be used as a precardiac catheterization screen. It provides assessment of congenital and acquired cardiovascular lesions and monitors the effects of therapy.

Premedication: Younger and uncooperative children may require sedation to remain still during the interval between injection and imaging. The sedative should be administered intramuscularly 30 minutes before the scan. A blocking agent (oral potassium perchlorate) is administered 1 hour before injection of the radionuclide.

Diet: The sedated child should be kept NPO for 4 hours before the procedure to prevent possible vomiting and aspiration of gastric contents.

Consent: An authorization signed by the parent or guardian is necessary.

Time: 5 minutes.

Procedure: An intravenous line is started in an upper extremity before the procedure to permit the injection of the radionuclide. Starting the IV in advance prevents the child from crying and the resultant Valsalva maneuver during administration of the drug that may impede the bolus or reverse certain shunts (1).

The child is placed in a sitting position and the gamma camera is positioned close to him over the precordium. Infants and very young children are studied in the supine position. The radionuclide is injected in the form of a bolus and is traced as it traverses the heart and great vessels. ^{99m}Tc-labeled pertechnetate or albumin are frequently used radiopharmaceuticals.

Preparation: (See section on "Brain Scan.") The only discomfort associated with this procedure will be during the venipuncture. Oral potassium perchlorate is administered to block the uptake of technetium by the thyroid gland.

Restraint Necessary: (See section on "Brain Scan.")

Aftercare: No physical aftercare is necessary.

RENAL IMAGING

Radionuclide renal imaging procedures provide information about kidney structure, function, and blood supply. Radionuclide imaging offers an alternative to radiographic studies if the patient is hypersensitive to radiopaque contrast media.

Premedication: If ^{99m}Tc is to be used, a blocking agent is administered 1 hour before the injection of the radionuclide (refer to Table 11-1).

Diet: No dietary restriction is necessary.

Consent: An authorization signed by the parent or guardian is necessary.

Time:

Renal Imaging: 30 minutes.

Radionuclide Cystography: 30 minutes.

Renogram: 30 minutes.

Procedure:

Renal Imaging: The radiopharmaceutical is injected intravenously and serial scintiscans are exposed for a 3- to 5-minute period for a total of 30 minutes. Delayed films several hours after injection may be necessary to visualize poorly functioning kidneys. The normal renal transit time of one of the most widely used radiopharmaceuticals, ^{131}I-Hippuran, is approximately 3 minutes. ^{99m}Tc-DTPA, a chelate-forming compound, is also commonly used.

Renogram: Renography provides a time-activity curve of the transit of a radionuclide through the kidney. Frequently used radiopharmaceuticals for this procedure are ^{131}I-Hippuran and ^{99m}Tc.
   The child is placed in a sitting position and the two scanning detectors are positioned near to the body over the kidneys. The radiopharmaceutical is injected intravenously and scanning is begun. Counts of radioactivity are recorded continuously on a strip count recorder (a device similar to that used to record an EKG) for approximately 20 minutes. Accurate placement of the scanning detectors is critical.

Radionuclide Cystography: This procedure is useful for the detection of vesicoureteral reflux. The child is placed in a supine position under the gamma camera and a bladder catheter is inserted. The radionuclide (usually ^{99m}Tc pertechnetate) in 5 ml of saline is instilled through the catheter. Scanning is begun immediately and serial scintiscans are exposed. When the child complains of an urge to void, the catheter is clamped and exposures are made while the child strains as if to void. The clamp is then removed and films are made during urination through the catheter. The catheter is then removed. Additional films are taken at 1-hour intervals as long as the radioactivity remains (1).

Preparation: (See section on "Brain Scan.") The child must drink a specified amount of liquid 30 minutes before the renogram. The actual amount of liquid varies among institutions. Adequate hydration is important, since dehydration may accentuate abnormalities, and overhydration may mask minimal abnormalities. If the child has had any x-ray procedures of the kidneys, the renogram must be delayed 24 hours. The child is encouraged to void immediately before the procedure.

Restraint Necessary: (See section on "Brain Scan".)

Aftercare: No physical aftercare is necessary.

THYROID STUDIES

Nuclear thyroid studies are noninvasive nuclear imaging procedures used to determine the size, position, and function of the thyroid gland. Thyroid scanning and thyroid uptake tests are used conservatively in pediatrics, since the juvenile thyroid gland is highly sensitive to radiation. In order to minimize radiation hazards, radiopharmaceuticals that depict the necessary information with a minimal radiation dose are used. These include iodine-123 and technetium pertechnetete (1).

Premedication: If ^{99m}Tc is to be used, a blocking agent is administered 1 hour before the injection of the radionuclide (refer to Table 11-1).

Diet: The child must be kept NPO 6 hours before a thyroid uptake study.

Consent: An authorization signed by the parent or guardian is necessary.

Time: 30 to 45 minutes.

Procedure:

Thyroid Scan: The radionuclide (^{99m}Tc) is administered intravenously. The child is positioned supine under the scanner with the neck hyperextended 20 minutes after injection. A pillow may be placed under the child's shoulders to hyperextend the neck. If a rectilinear scanner is used, the device passes laterally back and forth over the child's neck, making a soft clicking noise as it passes over the thyroid gland. The child is cautioned not to cough or swallow unless the scanner is to the side to minimize the motion of the thyroid gland. At the completion of the scan, the physician palpates the thyroid gland for the exact location of any thyroid nodules.

Thyroid Uptake Test: The radiopharmaceutical is administered (^{123}I is given orally and ^{99m}Tc intravenously). The child is placed in the same position as for a thyroid scan, and scanning is begun 20 minutes after the intravenous injection or 2 hours after the oral administration. The readings are taken periodically within the next 24 hours to measure the amount of radioactivity present in the thyroid. The radioactivity of the child's thigh may also be measured to correct for background radioactivity.

Preparation: (See section on "Brain Scan.") The child must not have taken any drugs that either contain iodine or that would block the thyroid from picking up the iodine, for example, adrenocorticosteroids, isoniazid, sulfonamides, or radiopaque materials. (Refer to the *Physician's Desk Reference* nuclear medicine supplement for a complete list.)

Restraint Necessary: (See section on "Brain Scan.")

Aftercare: No physical aftercare is necessary.

REFERENCES

1. James AE, Wagner HN, Cooke RE: *Pediatric Nuclear Medicine.* Philadelphia, WB Saunders Co, 1974.
2. Mandrillo MP: "Brain Scanning." *Nurs Clin North Am* 9(4):633, 1974.
3. Sodee DB, Early PJ: *Technology and Interpretation of Nuclear Medicine Procedures,* ed 2. St Louis, CV Mosby Co, 1975.
4. Handmaker H, Lowenstein JM: *Nuclear Medicine in Clinical Pediatrics.* New York, Society of Nuclear Medicine, 1975.
5. Early PJ, Razzack MA, Sodee DB: *Textbook of Nuclear Medicine Technology,* ed 2. St Louis, CV Mosby Co, 1975.

BIBLIOGRAPHY

Bronzino JD: *Technology for Patient Care.* St Louis, CV Mosby Co, 1977.
Conway JJ: "Radionuclide Imaging of the Central Nervous System in Children." *Radiol Clin North Am* 10(2):291, 1972.

Decker K, Backmund H: *Pediatric Neuroradiology.* Munich, Publishing Sciences Group, 1975.

Early PJ, Razzak MA, Sodee DB: *Textbook of Nuclear Medicine Technology,* ed 2. St Louis, CV Mosby Co, 1975.

Flitter HH: *An Introduction to Physics in Nursing,* ed 7. St Louis, CV Mosby Co, 1976.

Gelfand MJ, Silberstein EB: "Radionuclide Imaging, Use in Diagnosis of Osteomyelitis in Children." *JAMA* 237(3):245, 1977.

Goodwin PN, Roa DV: *An Introduction to the Physics of Nuclear Medicine.* Springfield, Ill, Charles C Thomas, 1977.

Handmaker H, Lowenstein JM: *Nuclear Medicine in Clinical Pediatrics.* New York, Society of Nuclear Medicine, 1975.

James AE, Wagner HN, Cooke RE: *Pediatric Nuclear Medicine.* Philadelphia, WB Saunders Co, 1974.

Nabdrukkim NO: "Brain Scanning." *Nurs Clin North Am* 9(4):633, 1974.

Sodee DB, Early PJ: *Technology and Interpretation of Nuclear Medicine Procedures, ed 2. St Louis, CV Mosby Co, 1975.*

APPENDIX A

Restraining Infants and Children for Diagnostic Procedures

The success of any pediatric diagnostic procedure depends largely on the skill with which the child is immobilized. Inadequate restraint not only makes a procedure more difficult for the examiner but also more dangerous for the child.

The reason for restraint should be explained to the parent and to the child. Small children often misinterpret restraint as part of the punishment received in a painful procedure, so every effort should be made to correct this misinterpretation.

The child's safety is of primary importance during immobilization. For this reason the assistant must keep careful watch on circulation of restrained extremities, the child's color, and his breathing pattern.

The following methods of restraint serve to immobilize the child for most of the procedures described in the preceding chapters.

Mummy Restraint (Fig. A-1)

1. Place a blanket or drawsheet flat on the examination table.
2. Place the infant supine on the sheet with the top of the sheet at the child's shoulderline and the bottom of the sheet extending 10 to 12 inches beyond his feet. Half the length of the sheet is left on one side and half on the other side.
3. Place the infant's arms in the anatomical position.
4. Fold half of the sheet snugly over the child's right arm, tucking the remainder underneath the trunk on the other side.

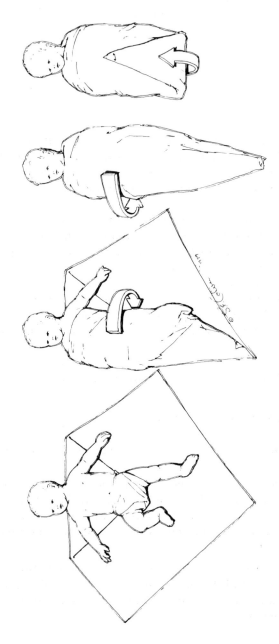

Figure A-1
Mummy restraint.

252

5. Bring the other half of the sheet over the child's body, tucking the end snugly behind his back.

6. Draw the bottom end of the sheet up, securing it with a safety pin.

(Some uses for this restraint: Scalp vein infusion; eye, ear, or throat examinations; nasogastric intubation.)

Restraint for Lumbar Puncture (Fig. A-2)

1. The child is placed on his side near the edge of the table. The head may be supported by a small pillow. The neck is flexed, the chin is brought close to the chest, and the knees are drawn up to the abdomen.

2. The assistant places one arm around the child's knees, grasping the wrists with the same hand. The assistant's other hand is placed around the back of the child's neck and shoulders. Flexion of the lumbar vertebrae

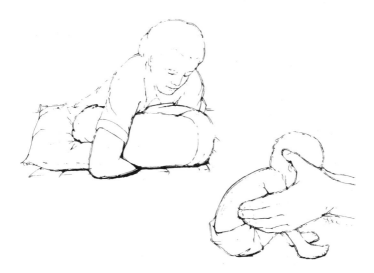

Figure A-2
Restraint for lumbar puncture.

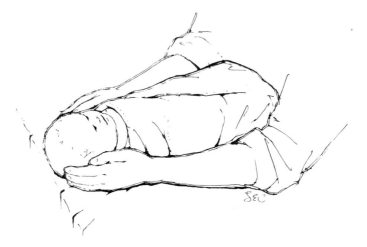

Figure A-3
Restraint for subdural tap.

may be enhanced by asking the child to arch his back "like a cat."

3. A final check on position is made. The child's back should be at the edge of the table, the pelvis and shoulders should be vertical to the floor, and the vertebral column should be aligned horizontal to the floor.

4. Throughout the procedure a close watch should be kept on the child's color and respiration. Flexion of a small infant's neck may occlude the airway.

5. The sitting position is preferable in small infants who have low cerebrospinal fluid pressure.

Restraint for Subdural Tap (Fig. A-3)

1. The child is secured with a mummy restraint.

2. He is placed in a supine position with the top of his head even with the edge of the examination table.

3. The assistant places his hands on either side of the child's head and holds the head firmly.

(Some uses for this restraint: Subdural tap, scalp vein infusion, eye examination.)

Clove Hitch (Fig. A-4)

1. Gauze or a diaper are used to form loops as shown in the illustration.
2. The loops are placed over the extremity to be restrained and adjusted snugly.
3. Adequate padding beneath the restraint is essential. Frequent checks (at least every 15 minutes) should be made for adequate circulation of the extremity.
4. If the child is restrained in bed, the restraints are secured to the mattress spring or bed frame, *never* to the side rails.

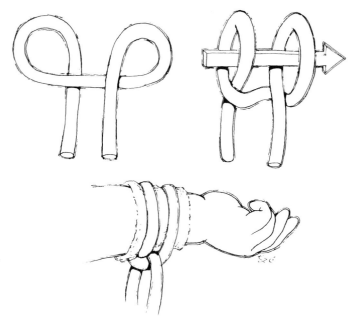

Figure A-4
Clove hitch.

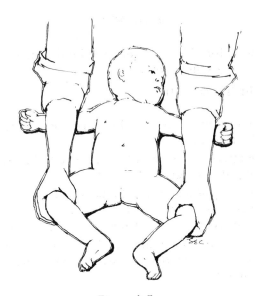

Figure A-5
Restraint for femoral venipuncture or suprapubic aspiration.

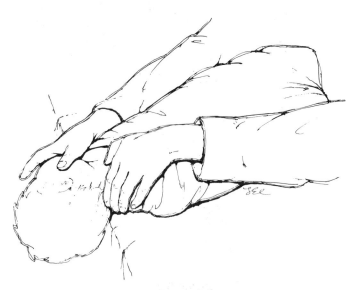

Figure A-6
Restraint for jugular venipuncture.

(Some uses for this restraint: Intravenous infusion or as a secondary restraint during a procedure while another portion of the body is immobilized.)

Restraint for Femoral Venipuncture or Suprapubic Aspiration (Fig. A-5)

1. The infant is placed supine with his legs spread apart. The assistant's hands are placed on the infant's knees as shown in the illustration.
2. For femoral venipuncture, a diaper may be placed over the infant's perineum to prevent possible contamination of the puncture site with urine.

Restraint for Jugular Venipuncture (Fig. A-6)

1. The child is secured with a mummy restraint.
2. The child's head is lowered over the side of the bed and held firmly by the assistant.

APPENDIX B
Normal Pediatric Laboratory Values

Table B-1
Hematology

Determination[a]	Age/Sex	Normal Range
Hematocrit (PVC)	Cord	50 – 60%
	Newborn	53 – 65
	Neonate	43 – 54
	Infant	30 – 40
	Child	31 – 43
	Thereafter: Male	42 – 52
	Female	37 – 47
Hemoglobin[b]	Cord	14 – 20 g/dl
	Newborn	15 – 22
	Neonate	11 – 20
	Infant	10 – 15
	Child	11 – 16
	Thereafter: Male	14 – 18
	Female	12 – 16
Fetal hemoglobin (HbF)	Newborn	40 – 70% of total
	Neonate	20 – 40
	Infant	2 – 10
	Thereafter	1 – 2

Table B-1
(Continued)

Determination[a]	Age/Sex		Normal Range
Nucleated red blood cell (nucleated RBC)	Cord		$250-500/mm^3$
	Day 1		$200-300$
	Day 2		$20-30$
	Thereafter		0
Osmotic fragility (fresh specimen) (50% hemolysis)			$0.42-0.46\%$ NaCl
Platelet count	Cord		$100-290\ 000/mm^3$
	Premature		$100-300,000$
	Newborn		$140-300,000$
	Neonate		$150-390,000$
	Infant		$200-473,000$
	Thereafter		$150-450,000$
Red blood cell count (RBC)	Newborn		$4.4-5.8\ ml/mm^3$
	Neonate		$4.1-6.4$
	Infant/child		$3.8-5.5$
	Thereafter:	Male	$4.7-6.1$
		Female	$4.2-5.4$
Blood indices			
MCH	Newborn		$32-34$ mg $(\mu\mu g)$
	Thereafter:	Male	$27-31$
		Female	$27-31$
MCV	Newborn		$96-108$ fl (μ^3)
	Thereafter:	Male	$80-94$
		Female	$81-99$
MCHC	Newborn		$32-33\%$

	Thereafter:	Male	32–36
		Female	32–36

Reticulocyte count		
Cord		3.0–7.0% total RBC
Newborn		1.1–4.5
Neonate		0.1–1.5
Infant		0.5–3.1
Thereafter		0.0–2.0

Sedimentation rate (ESR) (uncorrected)			
Newborn			0–2 mm/hr
Neonate/child			3–13
Thereafter:	Male	< 40 yrs	1–15
		> 40 yrs	1–20
	Female	< 40 yrs	1–20
		> 40 yrs	1–30

White blood cell count (WBC)[c]	Total mm^3	$\overline{X}\%$ Neutrophils	$\overline{X}\%$ Lymphocytes
Newborn	9000–30,000	61	31
1 week	5000–21,000	45	41
4 weeks	5000–19,500	35	56
6–12 months	6000–17,500	32	61
2 years	6200–17,000	33	59
Child/adult	4800–10,800	60	30

SOURCE: Reprinted with permission from Vaughn, V. C., McKay, R. J. and Behrman, R. E. (Eds.): *Textbook of Pediatrics*, ed. 11, Philadelphia, W. B. Saunders Co., 1979.

[a]Whole blood unless otherwise indicated.

[b]During the neonatal period, hemoglobin measurements from capillary blood are 2 – 3 g/dl greater than those in blood obtained by venipuncture.

[c]Eosinophilia (up to 20% of white blood cell count) may occur normally in infancy.

Table B-2
Chemistry

Determination	Specimen	Age/Sex	Normal Value
Acetone	Serum/plasma		
Qualitative			Negative
Quantitative (acetone and acetoacetic acid)			0.3 – 3.0 mg/dl
Albumin (See "Electrophoresis, protein")			
Aldolase (fructose-1.6-diphosphate; 37°C)	Serum	Infant	1.5 – 18.8 U/l
		Child	2.3 – 13.5
		Adult	1.5 – 12.0
Ammonia	Whole blood	Premature/jaundiced infant	100 – 200 g/dl
		Newborn	90 – 150
		Child	40 – 80
		Thereafter	40 – 110 (Conway method)
			40 – 80 (Enzymatic method)
Amylase (Amylochrome; 37°C)	Serum		45 – 200 dye units/dl
	Urine, 24 hours		40 – 330 dye units/hr

Test	Specimen	Category	Premature (mg/dl)	Full-term (mg/dl)
Ascorbic acid	Serum		0.6–2.0 mg/dl	
Base excess	Whole blood	Newborn	(–10)–(–2) mmol1/1	
		Infant	(–7)–(–1)	
		Child	(–4)–(+2)	
		Thereafter	(–3)–(+3)	
Bilirubin, direct (conjugated)	Serum		0.0–0.2 mg/dl	
Bilirubin, total	Serum	Cord	< 2	< 2
		0–1 day	< 8	< 6
		1–2 days	< 12	< 8
		3–5 days	< 16	< 12
		5–10 days	< 2	0.2–1.0
		Thereafter	< 2	0.2–1.0
Bromosulfophthalein (BSP; 5mg/kg)	Serum		< 10% at 30 min	
			< 5% at 45 min	
Calcium, ionized	Serum		4.5–5.2 mg/dl	
Calcium, total	Serum	Cord	8.2–11.1 mg/dl	
		Premature (1 week)	6.1–11.0	
		Newborn	5.9–10.7	
		Infant	9.0–11.0	
		Child	8.8–10.8	
		Thereafter	8.5–10.4	
		Cord	2.05–2.77 mmol/1	

Determination	Specimen	Age/Sex	Normal Value
		Premature (1 week)	1.53 – 2.75
		Newborn	1.48 – 2.68
		Infant	2.25 – 2.75
		Child	2.20 – 2.70
		Thereafter	2.13 – 2.60
	Urine, 24 hours		50 – 150 mg/d (diet-dependent)
Carbon dioxide, partial pressure, pCO_2	Whole blood, arterial	Newborn	27 – 40 mmHg
		Infant	27 – 41
		Male	35 – 45
		Female	32 – 45
Carbon dioxide (total CO_2)	Serum, venous	Cord	14 – 22 mmol 1/1 (arterial is approx. 2 mmol/1 lower)
		Premature (1 week)	14 – 27
		Newborn	17 – 24
		Infant	20 – 28
		Child	20 – 28
		Thereafter	23 – 29
Chloride	Serum	Cord	96 – 104 mmol/1
		Premature	95 – 110
		Newborn	96 – 107
		Thereafter	98 – 106
	Urine	Infant	2 – 10 mmol/d (diet-dependent)
		Child	15 – 40
		Thereafter	110 – 250

Analyte	Specimen		Reference range
	Urine, random		10–80 mmol/1 (normal diet)
	Sweat	Normal	0–30 mmol/1
		Marginal (e.g., asthma, Addison's disease, malnutrition, etc.)	30–70
		Cystic fibrosis	60–200
Cholesterol, total	Serum	Cord	45–100 mg/dl
		Newborn	45–150
		Infant	70–175
		Child	120–200
		Adolescent	120–210
		Thereafter	140–250
Cortisol	Plasma	8 AM specimen	6–25 g/dl (fluorometric)
			5–20 (RIA)
		4 PM specimen	2–18 (fluorometric)
			5–12 (RIA)
Creatine	Serum/plasma	Adult: Male	0.2–0.6 mg/dl
		Female	0.4–0.9
	Urine	Adult: Male	0–40 mg/d
		Female	0–80
Creatine kinase, CK (creatine phosphokinase, CPK; 30°C)	Serum	Newborn	10–300 U/l
		Adult: Male	12–65
		Female	10–50 (higher in blacks; lower at bed rest)

Table B-2
(Continued)

Determination	Specimen	Age/Sex		Normal Value
Creatinine	Serum	Cord		0.6 – 1.2 mg/dl
		Infant		0.2 – 0.4
		Child		0.3 – 0.7
		Adolescent		0.5 – 1.0
		Adult:	Male	0.6 – 1.2
			Female	0.5 – 1.1
	Urine	Infant		8 – 20 mg/kg/d
		Child		8 – 22
		Adolescent		8 – 30
		Adult		14 – 26
Creatinine clearance (endogenous)[a]	Serum and timed urine	Newborn		40 – 65ml/min/1.73 m²
		Child:	Male	98 – 150
			Female	95 – 125
		Adult:	Male	90 – 130
			Female	80 – 120
Disaccharide tolerance (dose: twice oral GTT dose)	Serum			20 mg/dl change in glucose concentration
Electrophoresis, protein (cellulose acetate)	Serum			

	Total Protein	Albumin	α_1-glob	α_2-glob	β-glob	γ-glob
Premature	4.3 – 7.6	3.1 – 4.2	0.1 – 0.5	0.3 – 0.7	0.3 – 1.2	0.3 – 1.4g/dl
Newborn	4.6 – 7.4	3.6 – 5.4	0.1 – 0.3	0.3 – 0.5	0.2 – 0.6	0.2 – 1.0
Infant	6.1 – 6.7	4.4 – 5.3	0.2 – 0.4	0.5 – 0.8	0.5 – 0.8	0.3 – 1.2
Thereafter	6.0 – 8.0[b]	3.5 – 4.7[c]	0.2 – 0.3	0.4 – 0.9	0.5 – 1.1	0.7 – 1.2[d]

Analyte	Specimen	Age	Value
Fatty acids	Serum		0.3 – 0.9 mmol/l
Fibrinogen	Plasma		125 – 300 mg/dl
			150 – 450
Folate	Serum	Newborn	6 – 13 ng/dl
		Thereafter	6 – 16
Galactose	Blood	Newborn/ Infant	0 – 20 mg/dl
Glucose, fasting	Serum/plasma	Cord	45 – 96 mg/dl
(glucose oxidase or		Premature[e]	20 – 60
hexokinase		Neonate[e]	30 – 60
method)		Newborn (1 day)	40 – 60
		Newborn	50 – 80
		Child	60 – 100
		Thereafter	70 – 105
	Blood	Thereafter	65 – 100
	Urine	Thereafter	0.5 – 1.5 g/d

Glucose tolerance Plasma (values in mg/dl)

Dosages		Time	Normal	Latent Diabetic	Diabetic
0 – 18 mo	2.5 g/kg	Fasting	65 – 105	105 – 120	> 120
18 mo – 3 yr	2.0	60 min	120 – 160	160 – 195	> 195
3 – 12 yr	1.75	90 min	100 – 140	140 – 150	> 150
> 12 yr	1.25 (max 100 g)	120 min	65 – 120	120 – 140	> 140
Adult	100 g total dose	180 min	65 – 105	105 – 120	> 120
		240 min	65 – 105	65 – 105	> 105
	Urine		no glycosuria	2 + to 4 + glycosuria on 1 – 2 spec	2 + to 4 + glycosuria on 2 or more spec

Table B-2
(Continued)

Determination	Specimen	Age/Sex	Normal Value			
			IgG (mg/dl)	IgM (mg/dl)	IgA (mg/dl)	Total γ (mg/dl)
Hemoglobin	Serum		0–3 mg/dl			
Immunoglobulin levels	Serum	Newborn	831–1231	6–16	0–5	843–1245
		1–3 mon	311–549	19–41	8–34	354–608
		4–6 mon	241–613	26–60	10–46	294–702
		7–12 mon	442–880	31–77	19–55	510–994
		13–25 mon	553–971	27–73	26–74	612–1128
		26–36 mon	709–1075	42–80	34–108	819–1229
		3–5 yr	701–1257	38–74	66–120	833–1323
		6–8 yr	667–1179	40–90	79–169	819–1405
		9–11 yr	889–1359	46–112	71–191	1080–1588
		12–16 yr	822–1170	39–79	85–211	984–1322
		Adult	853–1563	72–126	139–261	1104–1810
Iron-binding capacity	Serum	Newborn		60–175	g/dl	
		Infant		100–400		
		Thereafter		250–400		
		Elderly		200–300		
Iron, total	Serum	Newborn		100–250	g/dl	
		Infant		40–100		
		Child		50–120		
		Adult: Male		60–150		
		Female		50–130		
		Elderly		40–80		

		Total	Alpha	Beta	Chylo
Lactose tolerance test (Dosages: 0 – 2 yr, 3 g/kg; 2 – 10 yr, 2.5 g/kg; older children and adults, 2 g/kg [max of 100 g])	Plasma	Similar to GTT curve of same patient (disaccharide absorption impairment, little or no rise in sugar level)			
Lipase (olive oil, 37°C)	Serum	Infant 9 – 105 U/l Thereafter 20 – 180			
	Drainage duodenal	8 – 35			
Lipids, total	Serum	Newborn – 2 years 170 – 450 mg/dl 2 – 14 years 490 – 1000 Thereafter 400 – 800			
Lipoproteins	Plasma	Newborn 170 – 440	70 – 180	50 – 160	50 – 110mg/dl
		Infant 240 – 800	80 – 280	120 – 450	50 – 250
		Thereafter 500 – 1100	150 – 330	225 – 540	100 – 270
Osmolality	Serum	289 – mOsm/kg			
Osmolarity	Serum	270 – 285 mOsm/l			
	Urine	Infant 50 – 600 mOsm/l or mOsm/kg Child/adult 50 – 1400			
Oxygen capacity	Whole blood, arterial	1.34 ml/g hemoglobin			

Table B-2
(Continued)

Determination	Specimen	Age/Sex	Normal Value
Oxygen content	Whole blood, arterial		15 – 23 vol%
Oxygen pressure (pO₂)	Whole blood, arterial	Newborn	65 – 80 mmHg
		Thereafter	83 – 108 decreases with age
Oxygen, % saturation	Whole blood, arterial	Newborn	40 – 90%
		Thereafter	95 – 98
	Whole blood, venous	Newborn	30 – 80
		Thereafter	55 – 85
P₅₀[pO₂(0.5)]	Whole blood, arterial	Newborn	18 – 24 mmHg
		Thereafter	25 – 29
pH (37°C)	Whole blood, arterial	Premature (48 hours)	7.35 – 7.50
		Newborn	7.25 – 7.47
		Thereafter	7.33 – 7.43
	Whole blood, venous		7.33 – 7.43
Phenylalanine	Serum	Premature/low birth weight	2.0 – 7.5 mg/dl
		Full-term newborn	1.2 – 3.4
		Thereafter	0.8 – 1.8
Phosphatase, acid (phenylphosphate; 30°C)	Serum	Newborn – 2 weeks	10.4 – 16.4 KA/U/ml
		2 weeks – 13 years	8.6 – 12.6

Analyte	Specimen	Category	Reference range
Phosphatase, alkaline (p-nitrophenyl-phosphate, carbonate buffer; 30°C)		Thereafter: Male	0.5 – 11.0
		Female	0.2 – 9.5
		Newborn	50 – 165 U/l
		Child	20 – 150
		Thereafter	20 – 70
Phosphorus, inorganic	Serum	Cord	3.7 – 8.1 mg/dl
		Premature (1 week)	5.4 – 10.9
		Newborn	3.5 – 8.6
		Infant	4.5 – 6.7
		Child	4.5 – 5.5
		Thereafter	3.0 – 4.5 g/d
Potassium	Serum/plasma	Premature (cord)	5.0 – 10.2 mmol/1
		Premature (48 hours)	3.0 – 6.0
		Newborn (cord)	5.6 – 12.0
		Newborn	3.7 – 5.0
		Infant	4.1 – 5.3
		Child	3.4 – 4.7
		Thereafter	3.5 – 5.3
Protein-bound iodine (PBI)	Serum		4.0 – 8.0 µg/dl

Table B-2
(Continued)

Determination	Specimen	Age/Sex	Normal Value
Protein, total	Serum	Premature	4.3 – 7.6 g/dl
		Newborn	4.6 – 7.6
		Child	6.2 – 8.0
		Thereafter	6.0 – 8.0
	Urine, 24 hours		50 – 150 mg/d
	Urine first AM		< 20
	Urine, random		< 10
Sodium	Serum	Premature (cord)	116 – 140 mmol/l
		Premature (48 hours)	128 – 140
		Newborn (cord)	126 – 166
		Newborn	134 – 144
		Infant	139 – 146
		Child	138 – 145
		Thereafter	135 – 148 (diet-dependent)
Urea nitrogen	Serum/plasma	Cord	21 – 40 mg/dl
		Premature (1 week)	3 – 25
		Newborn	4 – 18

Analyte	Specimen	Category	Reference value
Uric acid	Serum/plasma	Infant/child	5 – 18
		Thereafter	7 – 18 (higher with high-protein diet)
		Child	2.0 – 5.5 mg/dl
		Thereafter: Male	3.5 – 7.2
		Female	2.6 – 6.0
	Urine		250 – 750 mg/day (lower with low purine diet)
Urobilinogen	Urine		0.5 – 3.5 mg/d
			0.5 – 4.0 EU/d
Vitamin A	Serum	Newborn	35 – 75 g/dl
		Child	60 – 100
		Thereafter	30 – 65
Vitamin B_{12}	Serum	Newborn	580 – 1140 pg/ml
		Thereafter	200 – 900
Vitamin C	Plasma		0.6 – 2.0 mg/dl
Vitamin E (tocopherols)	Serum		5 – 20 g/ml
Volume	Whole blood	Premature	90 – 108 nk.jg
		Newborn	80 – 110
		Infant	70 – 112
		Adult	72 – 100
	Plasma	Adult	49 – 59
	Urine	Newborn/Neonatal	50 – 300 ml/d

Table B-2
(Continued)

Determination	Specimen	Age/Sex	Normal Value
		Infant	350–550
		Child	500–700
		Adolescent	700–1400
		Thereafter: Male	800–2000
		Female	800–1600
	Gastric residue		20–100 ml (12-hour fasting)

SOURCE: Reprinted with permission from Vaughn, V. C., McKay, R. J., and Behrman, R. E. (Eds): *Textbook of pediatrics*, ed. 11, Philadelphia, W. B. Saunders Co., 1979.

[a]Endogenous creatinine clearance is expressed in milliliters per minute and is corrected to average adult surface area or 1.73 m²:

$$\frac{UV}{P} \times \frac{1.73}{A} = ml/min$$

where U = urine creatinine in mg/ml; P = plasma or serum creatinine in mg/ml; V = urine volume in ml/min; and A = estimated surface area in m².

[b]0–0.5 g higher in ambulatory individual.

[c]0–0.3 g higher in ambulatory individual.

[d]Up to 1.5 g/dl in blacks.

[e]While values as low as 20 mg/dl at birth are observed in seemingly normal newborns, parental glucose is usually administered when blood glucose level is less than 50 mg/dl.

[f]0.5 g/dl higher in ambulatory individuals; 0.2–0.4 g/dl higher in plasma.

Table B-3
Serology

Determination[a]	Titer/Interpretation
Antistreptolysin O titer (ASO)	
Normal	< 166 Todd units
Recent strep infection[b]	200–2500
Antihyaluronidase titer (AHT)	< 1:256
Cold agglutinins	0–1:32
C-reactive protein (CRP)	None detected
Cytomegalovirus (CMV)[c] (congenital CMV infection)[d]	≤ 1:32 indicates past or early infection
	≥ 1:64 may indicate past infection or early disease. A second specimen (4 – weeks) is needed for interpretation. IgM-specific antibody may be used to diagnose recent disease or congenital disease in the young infant.
Febrile agglutinins	
Typhoid O[e]	0–1:40
Typhoid H[e]	0–1:20
Brucella	0–1:20

Table B-3
(Continued)

Determination[a]	Titer/Interpretation
Rickettsia (Proteus OX 19, OX 2, OX K)	0 – 1:40
Tularemia	0 – 1:40
Hepatitis-associated (Australia) antigen (HB$_s$Ag)	None detected
Herpesvirus hominis (HVH)[c] (perinatal HVH infection)[f]	≤ 1:32 associated with previous or early infection
	≥ 1:64 may indicate recent infection. Repeat serum testing in 4 – 6 weeks would be required for proper interpretation
Heterophile antibody (mono "spot" test)	Negative
Rubella[g] (congenital)[h]	≥ 1:8 indicates previous infection and is generally considered to be protective for reinfection
Thyroid autoantibodies	
Thyroglobulin antibody (tanned red cell method)	< 1:10

SOURCE: Reprinted with permission from Vaughn, V. C., McKay, R. J., and Behrman, R. E. (Eds.): *Textbook of Pediatrics*, ed. 11, Philadelphia, W. B. Saunders Co., 1979.

[a]Serum unless otherwise indicated.

[b]Convalescent specimen should be examined to demonstrate rise in titer.

[c]Complement fixation method.

[d]Congenital CMV infection can be confirmed in the neonate by demonstrating IgM-specific CMV antibody. Cord serum or serum collected in the first month of life from the infant with symptomatic CMV infection usually has CMV antibodies equal to or greater than the mother's titer. This titer may decline, then persist beyond 6 to 8 months of age when maternal antibody would have diminished or disappeared.

[e]May be higher in individuals who have received typhoid vaccine.

[f]The presence of specific HVH IgM or the persistence of antibody beyond the time when passively acquired maternal antibody should have disappeared would confirm a perinatal infection.

[g]Hemagglutination inhibition method.

[h]Congenital rubella infection can be confirmed in the neonate by demonstrating the presence of rubella-specific IgM antibody. Maternal antibody (IgG) normally disappears from the infant's blood by 6 months of age. Therefore, persistence of rubella HI antibodies beyond 6 months or elevation of the titer beyond that of the mother is highly suggestive of congenital infection. After 12 months of age the possibility of postnatally acquired disease makes interpretation of a titer for determining congenital infection difficult.

Table B-4
Coagulation[a]

Determination	Specimen	Age	Normal Range
Activated clotting time (ACT) done at bedside	Hand held		1 min 50 sec. − 2 min 30 sec.
	Water bath		1 min 30 sec. − 2 min 10 sec.
Bleeding time (Ivy) (bedside)		Premature/newborn	1–8 min
Clot retraction		Thereafter	1–6
Clotting time (L-W)			40–94% at 2 hr
2 tubes	Whole blood		5–8 min
3 tubes	Whole blood		6–16
Fibrin split products	Serum		< 10 μg/ml
Fibrinogen	Plasma	Cord	216 mg/dl
		Newborn	125–300
		Thereafter	200–450
Fibrinolysin	Plasma		No lysis of clot in 2 hr
Partial thromboplastin time (PTT)[b]	Plasma	Premature	< 120 sec
	Plasma	Newborn	< 90

Prothrombin time, one stage (PT)[b]	Plasma	Thereafter	24–40
		Newborn	< 17 sec
		Thereafter	11–14
Thrombin time	Plasma		< 17 sec
Thromboplastin generation time (TGT)[b]	Plasma	Premature	8–24 sec at 6 min tube
		Newborn	8–20
		Thereafter	8–16

SOURCE: Reprinted with permission from Vaughn, V. C., McKay, R. J., and Behrman, R. E. (Eds): *Textbook of Pediatrics*, ed. 11. Philadelphia, W. B. Saunders Co., 1979.

[a]Coagulation factors (I to XIV) are low in the newly born, rising to adult levels during the first months of life.

[b]Moderate deficiency of coagulation factors dependent on vitamin K (II, prothrombin; VII, proconvertin; IX, plasma thromboplastin component; X, Stuart-Prower factor) occurs during the first days of life. Values return to near-normal levels within 1 week. This deficiency may account for prolonged PTT, PT, and TGT during this period.

Table B-5
Urinalysis

Determination	Age/Sex	Clean catch, midstream[a]	Catheterization	Normal Range Suprapubic bladder Puncture
Addis count				
Leukocytes				< 10
Erythrocytes				< 5
Casts				Occasional hyaline
Colony count, colonies/ml urine (fresh specimen)				
	Infant/child	< 1000	100	0
	Thereafter	< 10,000	100	0
Microscopic				
Leukocytes		0–4 per high-power field		
Erythrocytes		rare per high-power field		
Casts		rare per high-power field		
Osmolarity	Premature/newborn	50–600 mOsm/1		
	Thereafter	50–1400		
	Thereafter	> 850 (after fluid restriction)		
pH	Newborn/neonate	5.0–7.0		
	Thereafter	4.8–7.8		

Protein			
Qualitative			Negative
Quantitative			10–100 mg/d (higher after strenuous exercise)
Specific gravity, random	Newborn/infant		1.001–1.020
	Thereafter		1.001–1.030
	Thereafter		> 1.025 (after fluid restriction)
Sugar, qualitative (including glucose)			Negative
Volume	Newborn/neonate		50–300 ml/d
	Infant		350–550
	Child		500–1000
	Adolescent		700–1400
	Thereafter:	Male	800–2000
		Female	800–1600

SOURCE: Reprinted with permission from Vaughn, V. C., McKay, R. J., and Behrman, R. E. (Eds): *Textbook of Pediatrics*, ed. 11. W. B. Saunders Co., 1979.

aPure cultures with colony counts >100,000 are considered diagnostic in adults, whereas colony counts of >10,000 are usually considered diagnostic in children. Intermediate counts must be interpreted relative to the clinical situation. For females, the physician must be aware of the cleanliness and care used in collecting the specimen. Urine obtained by means of a plastic collection device or by voiding into a container without the prior preparation of the patient is usually contaminated and has limited usefulness in evaluating the possibility of urinary tract infections.

Table B-6
Cerebrospinal Fluid

Amount in the newborn	Up to 5 ml
Increases with age to adult figure	100 – 150 ml
Initial pressure	70 – 200 mmH$_2$O
pH	7.33 – 7.42
Appearance	Clear
Cell count (all lymphocytes, any polys in nontraumatic tap are abnormal)	
Under one year	Up to 10 cells/mm^3
1 – 4 years	Up to 8 cells/mm^3
Over 5 years	0 – 5 cells/mm^3
Glucose[a]	
6 months – 10 years	71 – 90 mg/100 ml
Over 10 years	50 – 80 mg/100 ml
Sodium	130 – 165 mEg/1
Potassium	2.8 – 4.1 mEg/1
Calcium	4.5 – 5.5 mg/100 ml
Magnesium	2.8 – 3.3 mg/100 ml
Chloride	
7 days – 3 months	108.8 – 122.5 mEg/1
4 – 12 months	112.7 – 128.5 mEg/1
13 months – 12 years	116.8 – 130.5 mEg/1
Specific gravity	1.005 – 1.009
Protein	
Ventricular fluid	6 – 15 mg/100 ml
Cisterna magna fluid	15 – 25 mg/100 ml
Lumbar CSF	20 – 45 mg/100 ml

[a]Usually, blood sugar level is obtained for comparison with CSF glucose level. The glucose level is less than, and varies proportionally with, the rise and fall of the plasma glucose level. Normal CSF glucose levels are about two-thirds the blood glucose level.

Table B-7

Radioisotopic Procedures

Determination	Specimen	Age	Normal Range
⁵¹Chromium			
Cell survival (T/2)	Whole blood		25–35 days/half-time
Red cell mass	Whole blood		28–32 mg/kg
⁵¹Chromium-albumin			
Normal	Urine		10–15% of dose/72 hr
Exudative enteropathy	Urine		6–12
Normal	Stool		0–1% of dose/72 hr
Exudative enteropathy	Stool		2–20
Rose bengal ¹³¹Iodine			
Normal	Urine		5–30% of dose/72 hr
Hepatocellular obstruction	Urine		10–20
Biliary obstruction	Urine		15–25
Normal	Stool		40–70% of dose/72 hr
Hepatocellular obstruction	Stool		10–50
Biliary obstruction	Stool		0–50
Schilling test (cyanocobalamine ⁵⁷Co)	Urine		10–40% of dose/24 hr
Thyroid uptake of ¹³¹I	Neck scan	Newborn	12–70% of dose/24 hr
		Neonate	8–50
		Infant	8–33
		Thereafter	7–25% of dose/6 hr
			8–33% of dose/24 hr
Thyroid uptake of ⁹⁹ᵐTcO₄	Neck scan		2.0–5.5% of dose within 20 min

SOURCE: Reprinted with permission from Vaughn, V. C., McKay, R. J., and Behrman, R. E. (Eds.): *Textbook of Pediatrics*, ed. 11, Philadelphia, W. B. Saunders Co., 1979.

285

Table B-8

Normal Values of Cellular Elements in Bone Marrow in Children Over 3 Months of Age

Elements	Range (%)
Myeloblasts	0−4
Myelocytes	7−25
Promyelocytes	0−6
Nonsegmented polymorphonuclear cells (including metamyelocytes)	7−30
Segmented polymorphonuclear cells	5−30
Eosinophils (all stages)	1−10
Monocytes	0−7
Lymphocytes	5−45
Nucleated red cells (principally normoblasts)	4−35
Megakaryocytes	$10-35/mm^3$
Total nucleated cell count	$100,000-200,000/mm^3$

Index